ANATOMY AND PHYSIOLOGY OF SPEECH LABORATORY TEXTBOOK

by

Harold M. Kaplan, Ph.D.

Visiting Professor, School of Medicine
Southern Illinois University

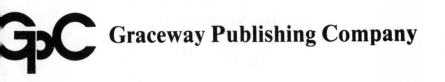 **Graceway Publishing Company**

Copyright © 1981 By Graceway Publishing Company

Manufactured in the United States of America

Library of Congress Catalog Card No.: 80-82927
ISBN 0-932126-04-9   Hardcover
ISBN 0-932126-05-7   Softcover

Published by:
Graceway Publishing Company
P.O. Box 159, Station "C"
Flushing, New York 11367

COLLABORATORS

CONTRIBUTOR TO SEVERAL EXERCISES

John G. Keene, M.D.
Memorial Hospital, Michigan City, Indiana

ILLUSTRATIONS

George F. Spiegel, M.S.
Southern Illinois University, Carbondale, Illinois

PREFACE

The text is directed toward students at any level needing introductory laboratory experience in anatomy and physiology, as part of their basic science education in speech pathology. The subject matter is thus generalized and the text can be supplementary to any of the relevant standard textbooks written for the general student. Many of the exercises included demand special expertise on the part of the instructor.

The work and the instrumentation involved are not intended to be at the level of sophistication attained by the experienced investigator in speech pathology. There is a great body of literature available to the research worker and clinician.

The writer has chosen exercises from those compiled in our laboratory for students in speech pathology. The 23 exercises listed actually cover 25 periods generally of two hours each. This permits adequate selection from a diverse pool for a one-semester course, commonly 17 weeks in length with one laboratory period per week. Most of the equipment and materials needed could be made available over a period of time. A laboratory designated for anatomy and physiology should be available. The prosected human cadaver requires access to a human anatomy laboratory.

Especial thanks are due Carol Gobleman and Janice Kuse at S.I.U. for their work in processing this manuscript.

Harold M. Kaplan

Table of Contents

Table of Contents

List of Figures

List of Figures

CHAPTER I
Anatomic Concepts

EXERCISE 1

GENERAL BODY COMPOSITION

OBJECTIVES

The beginner in speech pathology should learn anatomic terminology and appreciate at least in overview the structure of cells and
tissues which are building blocks of the body. The systems of the body
have a more immediate relevance to the speech function, but their
general organization is not dealt with in this brief laboratory exercise.

TIME REQUIRED

One and one-half laboratory periods - three hours. The time will
vary according to the selection of material by the staff.

MATERIALS

Compound light microscopes
Selected slides of cells and tissues
Slide projector and screen

Lens paper, methylene blue stain,
  iodine solution, ethanol, onions
Complete articulated human
  skeleton

DESCRIPTION

All descriptions of the body unless otherwise stated are referenced to a basic anatomic position. The person is upright with head facing forward and feet together. The upper extremities are fully dependent, the fingers extended, the palms facing forward and the thumbs abducted. A complete skeleton should be made available for the class. Determine from it the following relationships.

The median or midsaggital plane cuts the body into equal right and left halves. Planes parallel to the median plane are sagittal or parasagittal planes. The vertical planes perpendicular to the sagittal planes are frontal or coronal planes. A coronal plane cuts the body into front and back parts. Transverse planes section the body or appendages horizontally, making a cross section.

Anterior is equated with ventral, and posterior with dorsal. If a structure is ventral, it is in front. If a part is dorsal, it is in back. Superior, cranial, or cephalad structures are toward the head. In passing downward, the direction is caudal or inferior.

The sole of the foot is the plantar surface, and the upper surface is the dorsal surface. The volar or palmar surface of the hand refers to the palm; the dorsal or posterior surface of the hand refers to the back of the hand.

CELL and TISSUES

Cells

A cell is a minute mass of living substance, protoplasm, surrounded by a membrane. The governing area, or nucleus, is concerned with regulation of metabolism of the whole cell and also with cell division. The protoplasm of the cell exclusive of the nucleus is cytoplasm.

The microscopic structures in the cytoplasm are divided to organelles and inclusions. The organelles are the mitochondria, centrioles, fibrils and Golgi apparatus. The inclusions are aggregates of foods, pigments, granules and crystals.

Mitochondria are concerned with energy production. They contain enzymes which help transform foods into living protoplasm. The Golgi apparatus plays a part in secretory activity. Fibrils give stability to the cell. Centrioles are active during cell division. Figures 1-1 and 1-

2 illustrate a typical cell and representative cell types. The student should note that cells differ in form, size, appearance, chemical composition and activities.

FIGURE 1-1
GENERALIZED ANIMAL CELL

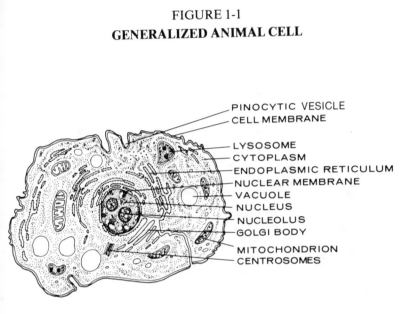

PINOCYTIC VESICLE
CELL MEMBRANE
LYSOSOME
CYTOPLASM
ENDOPLASMIC RETICULUM
NUCLEAR MEMBRANE
VACUOLE
NUCLEUS
NUCLEOLUS
GOLGI BODY
MITOCHONDRION
CENTROSOMES

Tissues

Cells aggregate to tissues. The basic tissues are epithelial, muscular, connective and nervous.

Epithelial tissues line internal and external surfaces. Epithelial cells protect the fluid environment within the body from the stresses of the external environment. These cells contain only enough intercellular material to cement the cells tightly together.

Connective tissues form the framework of the body. The subspecies which include tendons, ligaments, fascia, cartilage and bones are examples. They provide support, protection, and organization for the various pathways of communication, nutrition and innervation. Connective tissue cells are imbedded in an extensive matrix of intercellular material.Intercellular matrices include substances such as tissue fluid, various types of fibers, and the calcium deposits occurring in the matrix of bones. The types of cells, the matrix material and the geometry of the matrix provide keys for the classification of the sub-

FIGURE 1-2
REPRESENTATIVE CELL TYPES

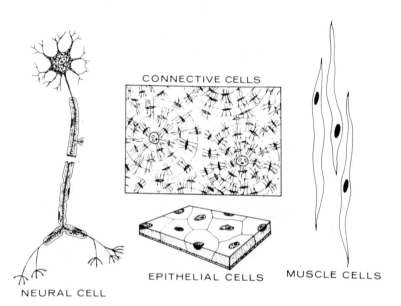

CONNECTIVE CELLS

EPITHELIAL CELLS   MUSCLE CELLS

NEURAL CELL

species of connective tissues.

Tendons are dense, fibrous cords or bands of variable length which connect a muscle with its movable bony or cartilaginous attachment. The fibers are composed of collagen and are arranged in parallel rows, with rows of cells called fibroblasts between the fibers.

Ligaments are bands or sheets of fibrous tissue connecting two or more bones, cartilages or other structures, or acting as a support for fasciae or muscles. The cells of ligaments are fibroblasts which lie between the fibers in rows.

Fasciae may be superficial or deep. Superficial fascia lies just under the skin and contains loosely arranged fibers interspersed with fat cells. Deep fascia is dense fibrous tissue investing all muscles, organs, blood vessels and nerves. In the speech organs, fascia binds adjacent structures together.

Cartilage (gristle) is firm, translucent connective tissue in which the amorphous intercellular substance exists as a firm jelly or gel. The matrix is composed of ordinarily invisible collagen fibers which form a dense network. The cells, called chondrocytes, lie in the matrix in little cavities called lacunae. A fibrous membrane called perichondrium covers cartilage. Blood vessels cannot enter the matrix, but substances can diffuse through the intercellular tissue fluid which is the bound water of the matrix gel. Cartilage is a common type of connective tissue in the speech organs.

Bone is a hard tissue consisting of cells in a matrix of ground substance and collagen fibers. The organic matrix is impregnated with minerals, especially calcium salts, which form about 67 per cent by weight of adult bone. Cells, called osteoblasts, lie in spaces called lacunae which are interconnected by small canals called canaliculi.In compact bone there is a system of larger canals mostly running lengthwise and containing small blood vessels. They are the haversian canals.The lacunae are usually arranged in concentric layers around the canals. The osteocytes within the lacunae send threads of protoplasm some distance along the radiating canaliculi. The canaliculi allow nutrients to pass from one cell to another and to and from the blood vessels in the haversian canals. Osteocytes produce and maintain the intercellular material. The bone as a whole functions for support, protection, production of all blood cells, and as a labile reservoir for calcium storage.

Nervous tissues provide the control and communication links for coordinating and integrating the activities of other tissues. Neural tissues are separated into the central nervous system consisting of the brain and spinal cord and the peripheral nervous system which includes the cranial and spinal nerves.

The propagated disturbance along a nerve is called a nerve impulse. Its nature is not fully understood, but it has an electrical concomitant called the action potential involving sodium, potassium and calcium interchanges between the exterior and interior of each selectively permeable nerve fiber membrane within the gross nerve trunk. The activity in one segment excites adjacent segments such that an all-or-none current sweeps from the nerve fibers to the effector structures.

The interval between any one nerve fiber and the several muscle fibers that it innervates is called the myoneural junction. Specialized electrochemistry within the cleft of the junction allows excitatory or inhibitory transmitters which are passed into the cleft from the nerve fibers to exert their effects on muscle cell membrane receptors on the other side. This results in muscle action potentials that excite complex chemical changes and contraction in the muscle.

Somewhat comparable junctions exist between nerve fibers proper which must link up in a chain fashion to transmit nerve impulses. These junctions are called synapses. The synaptic events between the presynaptic and postsynaptic terminals of such fibers importantly determine the basic nature and properties of neural conduction. The neurochemistry in junctions whether in brain, spinal cord, or peripheral nerves, must be known to the clinical neurologist.

Muscular tissue is contractile. Muscles pull and move or steady structures to which they are attached. The force is adjusted to the part the muscle has to play. In exerting a pull, a muscle sets up intrinsic forces that tend to change its shape, making it shorter and thicker. A muscle is elastic. This permits absorption of shock and makes the action smooth. There are three distinct types of muscle, smooth, cardiac and striated (skeletal). The first two are involuntary and are governed by autonomic nerves. The third is voluntary and governed by cerebrospinal (somatic) nerves. Speech structures involve voluntary muscles chiefly.

Smooth muscle cells are long and spindle-shaped. Each cell has one nucleus and many myofibrils which travel the length of the cell. The myofibrils are the contractile elements. Smooth muscles are typified by the blood vessels that occur in the speech structures.

Striated muscle has fibers which are much larger than those of smooth muscle. Each fiber has many nuclei and is covered with a sarcolemma. The fibers contain myofibrils that run the length of the cell. Each myofibril has alternating proteins, actin and myosin chiefly, along its length. The proteins give the appearance of bands running transversely across the myofibrils. This characteristic gives this tissue its name of striated, or striped muscle.

Fibers are bound into bundles by loose connective tissue. The bundles, in turn, are bound together to form a muscle. Each muscle at its more movable end, or insertion, acts through a tendon to move cartilage or bone.

PROCEDURE

HANDLE MICROSCOPES WITH EXTREME CARE. Microscopes are expensive and the delicate optics are easily damaged.

Care should be taken to avoid finger prints on the lenses. Use only lens tissue and lens cleaning fluids on the optical parts. The eyepiece(s) are removable; avoid letting them drop from the microscope. Oil immersion lenses will greatly enhance the resolution. Use the oil, however, only on the oil lens. Gently wipe off the excess oil from the lens after use. Then clean the lens with 100 per cent ethyl alcohol and dry it carefully with lintless lens paper.

Cells

1. Take a toothpick and gently scrape the inside of your cheek. Deposit the material on the toothpick onto a slide. Place a few drops of 95 per cent ethyl alcohol on the slide. Add 1-2 drops of methylene blue stain and cover with a coverslip.
   Under high power, identify and draw the following:

Cell	Nucleus	Nuclear Membrane
Vacuoles	Nucleolus	

   (NOTE: Methlylene blue stain is 10 gm of the powder with water to make up 100 ml of solution. The preparation of solutions is generally the responsibility of the technical staff.)
2. Slice a small piece of onion. Take one layer of onion skin from the inside of a ring. Place the layer of skin on a slide. Put a few drops of iodine solution on it. View the onion skin under low and high power. Draw and label a cell. Observe that plant cells have walls whereas animal cells have thin outer membranes.
   (NOTE: Iodine solution is 1 gm potassium iodide, 2 gm iodine, in 200 ml distilled water.)
3. Prepare a clean slide. Sterilize a finger with 70 per cent ethyl alcohol and prick the distal phalanx of the finger with a sterile disposable lancet. Put a drop of blood on the slide. Take a second slide and make a thin blood smear by bringing one edge of the second slide over the edge of the blood and then dragging the blood with the edge of the second slide in the opposite direction. Draw the unstained red cells under low and high power.

Stained human blood films, obtained from commercial biological supply houses, are consistently of good quality. These are relatively permanent and can be obtained and stored in quantity by the staff.

Tissues

Stained slides of tissues purchased from biologic supply houses should be available. The following is a suggested list:

> Nerve fiber, cerebral cortex, spinal cord, cochlea, artery, larynx, trachea, thryroid gland, skeletal muscle, smooth muscle, stratified squamous epithelium, glandular epithelium, simple columnar epithelium, tooth, tongue, skin, and hyaline cartilage.

The instructor can select slides from the list as time permits. Using a slide projector, it is advantageous to demonstrate the stained tissue sections prior to individual study. The student should then examine the material under increasing magnifications of a light microscope.

EXERCISE 2

THE HUMAN SKULL

OBJECTIVES

The soft anatomic structures for speech lie almost entirely in the head, neck and thorax and the framework of these regions needs to be understood. Exercises 2 and 3 permit a detailed study of the skull bones. All figures have been placed in Exercise 3.

TIME REQUIRED

Two laboratory periods for Exercise 2 - four hours. Overlap with the beginning of Exercise 3 is compatible if the time frame warrants it.

MATERIALS

Skeletons and intact skulls (with detachable calvaria)
Disarticulated cranial, facial and hyoid bones

Pipe cleaners or flexible pointers
Advanced, illustrated textbooks and atlases of anatomy

DESCRIPTION AND PROCEDURE

The skull bones include those of the cranium and those of the face. These will be studied at this point. Additional observations continue in Exercise 3. A practical method to undertake this study is to have one student read the descriptions herein while the other laboratory partners locate and identify the structures as read. Use a supplementary, advanced anatomy text and atlases. Locate structures on the skull with soft pointers (e.g. pipe cleaners) to avoid damage. Tabulate the bones which are paired and those which are unpaired.

Cranial Bones

The bones of the cranium are seen best, but not exclusively, in two views, norma verticalis and norma lateralis. The cranial bones include the frontal, parietal, occipital, temporal, sphenoid and ethmoid.

Examine in detail the superior aspect of the skull (norma verticalis). This consists of the dome-like portion of the cranium. The unpaired frontal bone is most anterior and forms the prominence of the forehead. Immediately posterior, the paired parietal bones cover most of the superior and lateral aspects of the cranium. The parietal bones are fused medially by an immovable articulation called a suture. Sutures belong to a class of immovable joints called synarthroses. All articulations between bones in the skull are synarthroses except the temporo-mandibular joint. The most posterior bone seen in the superior view is the unpaired occipital. It forms the back of the skull, or major portion of the occiput.

Examine in detail the lateral view of the skull (norma lateralis). This allows visualization particularly of the temporal and sphenoid bones. The paired temporal bones are marked externally by the external acoustic meatus and by the temporal process of the zygomatic arch which juts out laterally from the skull and extends anteriorly to fuse with the zygomatic process of the frontal bone. Each temporal bone is divided into squamous, petrous and tympanic parts. The squamous part consists of the large, thin plate which lies anteriorly and superiorly and articulates with the parietal and sphenoid bones. The petrous part includes the portion housing the inner ear and it lies between the sphenoid and occipital bones at the base of the skull. The tympanic part of the temporal bone houses the external acoustic meatus. It is inferior to the squama and anterior to the mastoid process.

The styloid process of the temporal bone is a variably long projection, pointing downward and forward from its origin at the inferior aspect of the temporal bone. The process is important in that it gives rise to muscles of the tongue and pharynx and also to ligaments that attach to the mandible and hyoid bone.

The mastoid process of the temporal bone is at the posterior part of that bone. Externally it gives attachment to many muscles. Internally it is hollowed out into air-sacs, or cells, which are diverticula of the tympanic antrum. The antrum is an irregular space which communicates with the tympanic cavity.

The sphenoid is a single bone extending across the lower front of the cranium from side to side. When disarticulated, its shape as seen in anterior view resembles that of a butterfly. The lateral processes of the sphenoid are "wings." The larger of these, the great wings, can be seen on either side anterior to the temporal bone. The interior of the skull (seen later) provides another view of the sphenoid. A saddle-shaped structure, the sella turcica which holds the pituitary gland, is the most prominent central part of the sphenoid, seen only in the internal view.

Examine in detail the anterior view of the skull (norma frontalis). Note the single ethmoid bone located inferior to the unpaired frontal bone and anterior to the sphenoid. The ethmoid forms part of the anterior aspect of the cranium and part of the eye socket (orbit). Observe that its descending, central perpendicular plate fuses at its base into the vomer bone. The vertical plate is the bony framework of the median septum of the nose. In the frontal (anterior) view, the plate is hidden in life by the presence of a large triangular wedge of cartilage anterior to it. It is also partly obscured anteriorly by the small, paired nasal bones.

In its most superior aspect the ethmoid bone presents right and left extensions, called labyrinths, which are thin-walled cellular cavities. This uppermost section is hidden internally within the anterior cranial fossa of the skull. It is seen only by removing the calvarium and looking into the anterior, interior floor from above. Note the projection of the ethmoid into the fossa as a prominence called the crista galli. The prominence is surrounded by a perforated plate which allows the olfactory nerve to pass from the nose to the forebrain.

Facial Skeleton

The bones of the face include the mandible, maxilla, nasal, zygomatic, inferior nasal concha, lacrimal, palatine and vomer. These are seen best in the frontal view (norma frontalis). These bones form the framework of the orbits, cheeks, nose and mouth. The hyoid bone will also be considered, but for convenience only, with this group.

The openings for the nasal passages (anterior nares) are formed by the paired maxillae (cheek bones) inferiorly and laterally. Superiorly the paired nasal bones comprise the external anterior aspect and bridge of the nose. The nasal septum is composed of both cranial and facial bones which include the vomer and the perpendicular plate of the ethmoid bone. The paired inferior conchae are sparate bones and are the largest of the three pairs.

The vomer is a median-placed bone in the floor of the nose, upon which the perpendicular plate of the ethmoid rests. The vomer constitutes the inferior and posterior aspects of the nasal septum. The borders of the vomer will also be seen to articulate with the sphenoid, palatine and maxillary bones. The posterior border of the vomer separates the posterior nares (choanae).

The mouth is bounded by facial bones. The palatine bones and the palatine processes of the maxillary bones form the roof of the mouth (hard palate). The mandible completes the inferior aspect of the mouth. In embryonic development, the paired maxillae fuse centrally and in their most anterior aspect a premaxillary bone is wedged in between them.

The maxillae on each side form the central aspect of the facial framework. Their medial aspects form the external lateral walls of the nose. The medial parts also form the floor of the nose, the floor of the orbits, and the alveolar processes which carry the upper teeth.

The body of each maxilla is hollowed out to a pyramidal space called the maxillary sinus (antrum of Highmore). This is the largest of the paranasal sinuses. It empties by small openings into the middle meatus of each nasal cavity (naris). The contribution of these sinuses to the resonance function of speech is probably very small. The floor of the maxillary sinus is just above the maxillary teeth. (Commercially cut skulls are available which allow the student to look into all the cavities within the skull.)

The cheeks are formed superiorly by the zygomatic bones as well as by the maxillary bones. The zygomatic bones form the prominence of the cheeks, part of the walls of the orbit, and some of the temporal and infratemporal fossae.

Examine the bones comprising the orbits. Each orbit is formed on its medial aspect, going from anterior to posterior, by the frontal process of the maxilla, the lacrimal bone, and the ethmoid bone. The roof contains the orbital plate of the frontal bone and the lesser wing of the sphenoid. The floor is composed of the orbital process of the zygomatic bone, the orbital surface of the maxilla, and to a small extent the palatine bone posteriorly. Laterally the zygomatic bone and the greater wing of the sphenoid complete the orbit. The apex of the orbit is most posterior and is formed by the optic foramen.

Examine the unpaired mandible. This bone shapes the chin and the angles of the lower jaw. The mandible is comprised of the body, which is a curved horizontal section, and the paired rami which unite with the ends of the body and extend almost vertically. Study the external and internal surfaces of the body of the mandible, noting the mental protuberance, mental foramen, mental spines and alveolar border.

Examine one ramus. This extends superiorly to articulate with the mandibular fossa of the temporal bone. The uppermost facet at the extremity of the ramus is the mandibular condyle. A semilunar notch in the upper border of each ramus separates the anterior coronoid process from the posterior condyloid process. The temporalis muscle inserts on the coronoid process. Other mandibular muscles are described in Exercise 4.

Mandibles from persons of different age groups should be made available, if possible. Compare these in form and general structure, noting the changes occurring over time. Relate changes to possible changes in speech function.

The articulation between the mandible and skull is the temporomandibular joint. This is the only movable joint (diathrosis) in the skull and, because of the complexity of its motions, it is subdivided into both a hinge (ginglymus) and gliding (arthrodial) joint.

The unpaired hyoid bone lies in the anterolateral aspect of the neck just superior to the thyroid cartilage of the larynx. It is U-shaped, having a central part, or body, which is in the anterior aspect of the upper neck, and a pair of extensions which project dorsally from either side of the body. These extensions are the greater cornua. At the junctions of the body and greater cornua there rise small eminences called the lesser cornua.

The hyoid bone is not a part of the skull. It is, however, connected to it by the paired stylohyoid ligaments which run from the paired styloid processes of the temporal bone to the apex of each lesser cornu. The hyoid bone connects inferiorly to the larynx by the single thyrohyoid ligament.

The hyoid serves to suspend the larynx and it also an area of attachment for several muscles which have to do with movements of the mandible, tongue and larynx.

EXERCISE 3

BONY STRUCTURES OF THE SKULL

OBJECTIVES

This Exercise continues the study of the skull. The student is asked at this point to examine in detail foramina, fossae, sutures, various processes and the paranasal sinuses.

TIME REQUIRED

Two laboratory periods - four hours

DESCRIPTION AND PROCEDURE

One student is to read the descriptions herein while others in the group are to locate and point out in detail the structures on the skull. (The student has probably by now realized that some of the nomenclature used here includes Latin (and some Greek) terms. The latinization is in agreement with the Nomina Anatomica adopted by the International Nomenclature Committee and the International Congress of Anatomists. For the most part, however, the English equivalent has been selected in the following descriptions.)

Sutures

Sutures of the skull are immovable joints, or synarthroses. The bones are separated only by a thin layer of fibrous tissue. Study all sutures described

The suture separating the frontal and parietal bones is the coronal suture. The suture between the parietal bones is the sagittal suture. The suture between the parietal and occipital bone is the lambdoidal suture. Other sutures are named for the part of a bone involved or for two bones involved. The squamosal, intermaxillary, zygomaticotemporal and sphenoparietal sutures are examples.

The lambda is the point where the sagittal suture meets the lambdoidal suture. The bregma is the point where the sagittal and coronal sutures unite.

Foramina

A foramen is an opening which transmits some soft structure. Thus, the foramen magnum is a large opening in the occipital bone on the base of the skull which provides an exit for the spinal cord. Table 3-1 summarizes the major skull foramina and their function. Locate and examine these foramina.

Fossae

A fossae is a depression. Study the fossae as described herein. In the anterior lateral part of the roof of the orbit, the lacrimal fossa holds the lacrimal gland. The anterior medial aspect of the orbital floor contains a fossa for the lacrimal sac.

The temporal and infratemporal fossae lie above and below the zygomatic arch, respectively. The temporal fossa is bounded above by the infratemporal crest, a ridge extending anteriorly from the root of the zygomatic arch on the temporal bone. The infratemporal fossa is bounded by the infratemporal crest, the zygomatic process of the maxilla, the great wing of the sphenoid, the lateral pterygoid plate, the articular tubercle of the temporal bone and the alveolar border of the maxilla. Just medial to the temporal root of the zygomatic arch note the mandibular fossa for the articulation of the mandible and the temporal bone. Medial to the mastoid process find the mastoid notch

FIGURE 3-1
LATERAL VIEW OF THE SKULL, NORMA LATERALIS

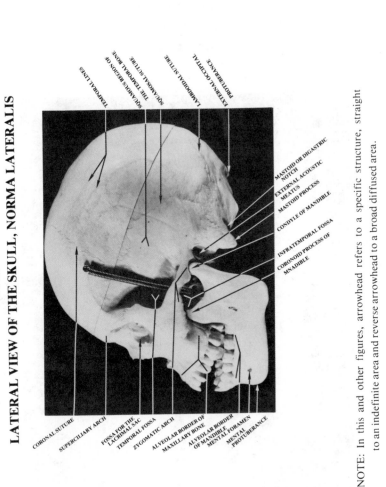

TEMPORAL LINES

SQUAMOUS REGION OF THE TEMPORAL BONE

SQUAMOSAL SUTURE

LAMBDOIDAL SUTURE

EXTERNAL OCCIPITAL PROTUBERANCE

MASTOID OR DIGASTRIC NOTCH

EXTERNAL ACOUSTIC MEATUS

MASTOID PROCESS

CONDYLE OF MANDIBLE

INFRATEMPORAL FOSSA

CORONOID PROCESS OF MNADIBLE

CORONAL SUTURE

SUPERCILIARY ARCH

FOSSA FOR THE LACRIMAL SAC

TEMPORAL FOSSA

ZYGOMATIC ARCH

ALVEOLAR BORDER OF MAXILLARY BONE

ALVEOLAR BORDER OF MANDIBLE

MENTAL FORAMEN

MENTAL PROTUBERANCE

NOTE: In this and other figures, arrowhead refers to a specific structure, straight to an indefinite area and reverse arrowhead to a broad diffused area.

or digastric fossa serving as the origin of the posterior belly of the digastric muscle.

In the base of the skull the jugular foramen cuts through the jugular fossa. Two pterygoid plates converge anteriorly to enclose the pterygoid fossa which holds the medial pterygoid and palatal tensor

FIGURE 3-2
UPPER ASPECT OF THE SKULL
NORMA VERTICALIS

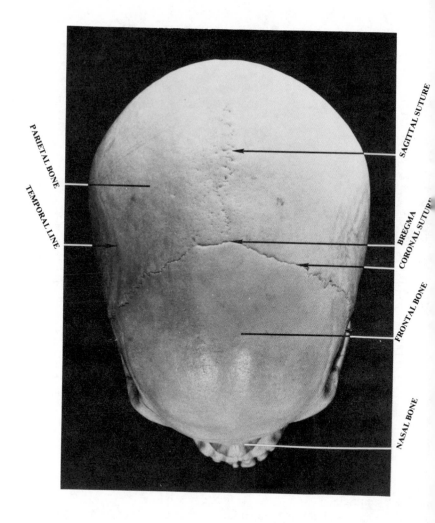

PARIETAL BONE

TEMPORAL LINE

SAGITTAL SUTURE

BREGMA

CORONAL SUTURE

FRONTAL BONE

NASAL BONE

TABLE 3-1
FORAMINA OF SKULL

Name	Location	Structure Transmitted
Magnum	Base occipital bone	Spinal cord
Jugular	Lateral to foramen magnum	Jugular vein; nerves IX, X, XI
Incisive	Anterior hard palate	Nasopalatine nerve and vessels
Greater Palatine	Lateral hard palate	Greater palatine nerve
Lesser Palatine	Lateral hard palate	Lesser palatine nerve & vessels
Ovale	Base of lateral pterygoid plate	Mandibular nerve
Spinosum	Posterior to foramen ovale	Middle meningeal vessels
Lacerum	Medial to foramen ovale	Closed by fibrocartilage of auditory tube
Mastoid	Posterior to mastoid process	Br. occipital a. to dura
Stylomastoid	Between mastoid process and styloid process	Facial nerve
Condyloid	Posterior to occipital condyle	Emissary vein
Hypoglossal canal	Anterior to occipital condyle	Hypoglossal nerve
Mental	Lateral mandible	Mental nerve and vessels
Infraorbital	Below orbit	Infraorbital nerve and vessels
Supraorbital	Above orbit	Supraorbital nerve and vessels
Optic	Apex of orbit	Optic nerve
Rotundum	Cerebral surface of great wing of sphenoid	Maxillary nerve
Pterygoid canal	Above medial pterygoid plate through sphenoid	Pterygoid nerve
Sphenopalatine	Formed by sphenoidal part of palatine and body of sphenoid	Pterygopalatine nerve and vessels
Pterygopalatine	Formed by articulation of vertical part of palatine and maxilla	Greater palatine nerve and vessels
Pharyngeal canal	Lateral to vaginal process on body of sphenoid	Pharyngeal nerve
Carotid canal	Anterior to jugular fossa	Internal carotid artery
External acoustic meatus	Lower exterior temporal bone	Sound waves
Internal acoustic meatus	Medial aspect petrous part of temporal bone	Facial and auditory nerves
Hiatus of facial	Anterior aspect petrous part	Greater petrosal nerve
Mandibular	Medial side ramus of mandible	Inferior alveolar nerve and vessels

(tensor veli palatini) muscles. The pterygopalatine fossa lies anterior to the great wing of the sphenoid and communicates with the infratemporal fossa via the pterygomaxillary fissure. It contains the maxillary nerve and the pterygopalatine ganglion. The foramen rotundum, sphenopalatine foramen, pterygoid canal, pharyngeal canal, and pterygopalatine canal all open into this space.

FIGURE 3-3
INFERIOR VIEW OF THE SKULL, NORMA BASALIS

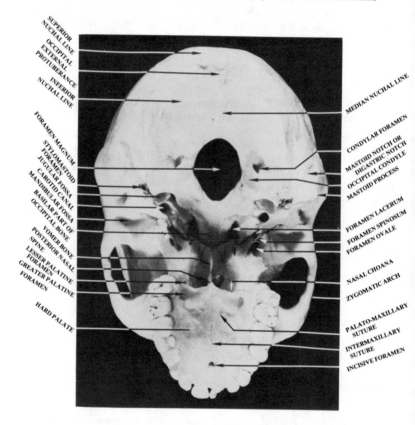

Remove the calvarium (upper skull plate) and examine the interior of the skull. Note that the internal skull base is divided into the anterior cranial fossa, middle cranial fossa and posterior cranial fossa.

The anterior fossa supports the frontal lobes of the cerebrum and contains several grooves. The chiasmatic groove extends from each optic foramen and provides space for the optic nerve and chiasm

FIGURE 3-4

NORMA BASALIS, OPENINGS OF THE CRANIUM

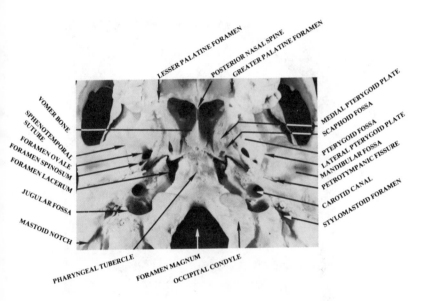

(decussation of optic tracts). Anteriorly, the olfactory grooves lie on either side of the crista galli and these grooves hold the olfactory bulbs which lie on the cribriform plate of the ethmoid bone.

The middle cranial fossa supports the temporal lobes of the cerebrum. The sella turcica is located therein, forming a saddle to seat the pituitary gland. A carotid groove lies on each side of the saddle.

The posterior cranial fossa, in the occipital region, holds the cerebellum, medulla oblongata and pons. The foramen magnum lies in its center.

Examine the fossae in the mandible, on the inner aspect of the bone. These fossae are named for the salivary glands. On either side of the mental spines, which are on the inner aspect of the mental symphysis, a shallow fossa is a recessed lodging for the sublingual salivary glands. These depressions are just superior to the mylohyoid line which runs posteriorly along the middle of the inner surface of the body of the

FIGURE 3-5
INTERIOR VIEW OF THE SKULL

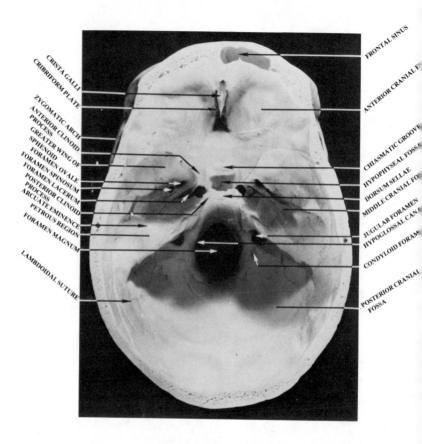

CRISTA GALLI
CRIBRIFORM PLATE
ZYGOMATIC ARCH
ANTERIOR CLINOID PROCESS
GREATER WING OF SPHENOID
FORAMEN OVALE
FORAMEN SPINOSUM
FORAMEN LACERUM
POSTERIOR CLINOID PROCESS
ARCUATE EMINENCE
PETROUS REGION
FORAMEN MAGNUM
LAMBDOIDAL SUTURE

FRONTAL SINUS
ANTERIOR CRANIAL F
CHIASMATIC GROOVE
HYPOPHYSEAL FOSS
HYPOPHYSEAL FOSSA
DORSUM SELLAE
MIDDLE CRANIAL FO
JUGULAR FORAMEN
HYPOGLOSSAL CAN
CONDYLOID FORAM
POSTERIOR CRANIAL FOSSA

mandible. Inferiorly, a slightly larger fossa lodges the submandibular gland.

Raised Structures

In the norma frontalis the paired superciliary arches are the prominences above the orbits. The arches provide attachment for the corrugator muscles. The mental protuberance (chin) is prominent. The middle and inferior nasal conchae are also visible in the frontal view.

FIGURE 3-6
INTERIOR OF SKULL, ENLARGED SECTION

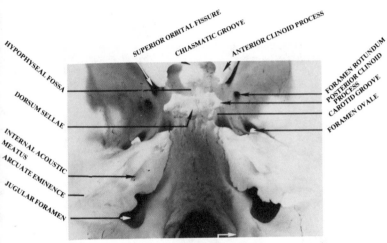

SUPERIOR ORBITAL FISSURE

CHIASMATIC GROOVE

ANTERIOR CLINOID PROCESS

HYPOPHYSEAL FOSSA

FORAMEN ROTUNDUM

POSTERIOR CLINOID PROCESS

CAROTID GROOVE

DORSUM SELLAE

FORAMEN OVALE

INTERNAL ACOUSTIC MEATUS

ARCUATE EMINENCE

JUGULAR FORAMEN

HYPOGLOSSAL CANAL

In the norma lateralis the zygomatic arch is a bony arch to the side of the orbit. It is composed of processes from the zygomatic and temporal bones which unite in a suture. The superficial and deep parts of the masseter muscle take origin from this arch and the temporalis muscle passes medial to it. Directly behind the arch is the infratemporal crest which separates the temporal fossa from the infratemporal fossa. The temporal lines visible on the external squamous part of the temporal bones are slight elevations marking the superior extent of the temporalis muscle.

Still in the lateral view, locate the mastoid and styloid processes, the former posterior and the latter inferior to the external auditory meatus. The mastoid process contains air cells and serves as a point of attachment for the posterior belly of the digastric, sternocleidomastoid and other muscles involved in movements of the head. The stylohyoid, styloglossus, and stylopharyngeus muscles arise from the styloid process.

In the norma basalis note that the pterygoid processes project into

FIGURE 3-7
ANTERIOR VIEW OF THE SKULL
(NORMA FRONTALIS)

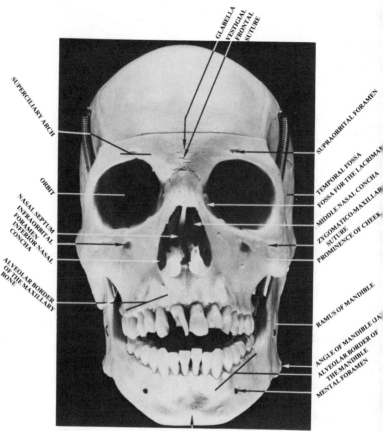

MENTAL PROTUBERANCE

the pharyngeal area to provide attachment for the pterygoid muscles. The process on each side is divided to a medial and lateral plate. Pterygoid muscles originate from the lateral plate and the superior pharyngeal constrictor attaches to the medial plate. A curved projection, the pterygoid hamulus, arises from the lower end of the medial plate and serves as a surface upon which the tendon of the palatal tensor (tensor palati) muscle glides.

As seen in the basal view, the broad occipital condyles allow articulation of the atlas with the occipital bone. The external occipital protuberance is a projection which is at the base of the skull posterior to the foramen magnum. It provides a connecting point for the nuchal ligament, a fibrous structure extending over the spines of the cervical vertebrae. The nuchal lines extend from the external occipital protuberance, indicating the attachments of neck and back muscles.

The pharyngeal tubercle and the posterior nasal spine are in the anterior part of the base of the skull. The pharyngeal tubercle, anterior to the foramen magnum on the basilar part of the occipital bone, gives rise to the fibrous raphe of the pharynx and to the superior pharyngeal constrictor muscle. Somewhat anterior and inferior, the posterior nasal spine projects from the middle of the posterior limit of the hard palate. It is composed of a small process from each of the palatine bones. The posterior nasal spine provides origin for the uvular muscles which insert into the uvula.

Turn again to the internal aspect of the skull, this time to view the raised structures therein. The crista galli and cribriform plate in the anterior fossa, the petrous part of the temporal bone separating the middle and posterior fossae, and the various parts of the sella turcica in the middle cranial fossa are most prominent.

The crista galli and cribriform plate have already been described. The perforated plate allows the olfactory nerves to pass from the nasal mucosa to the smell areas of the brain.

The auditory mechanism is in the petrous portion of the temporal bone. Note the petrous ridge in the internal aspect of the skull. The external auditory meatus allows access to the mechanism. A rounded area in the middle of the petrous region, the arcuate eminence (eminentia arcuata), marks the superior semicircular canal.

Examine the previously described sella turcica for its raised areas. The anterior, middle and posterior clinoid processes project along the sides of the saddle. The dorsum sellae forms the back of the saddle and the tuberculum sellae forms the front.

Miscellaneous Features

This category arbitrarily includes the paranasal sinuses, nasal septum and nasal choanae (posterior nares).

The paranasal sinuses consist of the frontal, ethmoid, sphenoid and maxillary sinuses. The sizes and shapes of these cavities vary among

FIGURE 3-8
FRONTAL BONE

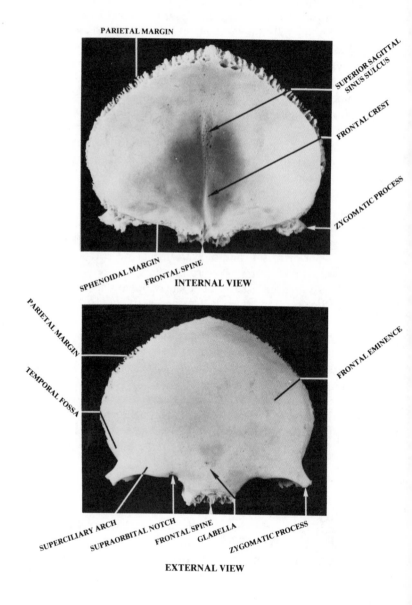

FIGURE 3-9
PARIETAL BONE

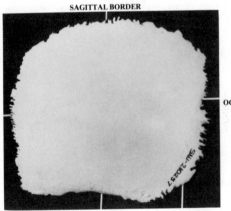

SAGITTAL BORDER

OCCIPITAL BORDER

FRONTAL BORDER

GROOVE FOR MENINGEAL VESSEL

SPHENOIDAL ANGLE

MASTOID ANGLE

TEMPORAL (SQUAMOUS) BORDER

INTERNAL SURFACE

LEFT ANTERIOR VIEW

SAGITTAL BORDER

OCCIPITAL BORDER

FRONTAL BORDER

TEMPORAL (SQUAMOUS) BORDER

MASTOID BONE

LEFT EXTERIOR VIEW

FIGURE 3-10
TEMPORAL BONE

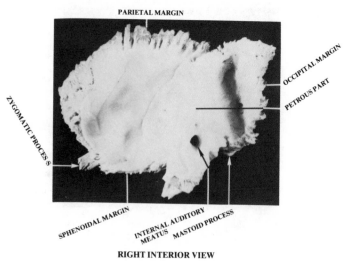

RIGHT INTERIOR VIEW

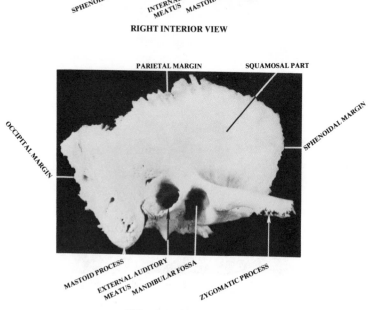

RIGHT EXTERIOR VIEW

FIGURE 3-11
OCCIPITAL BONE

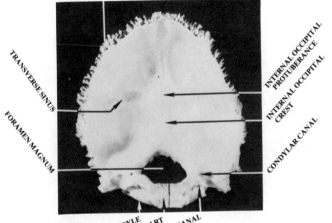

INTERNAL VIEW

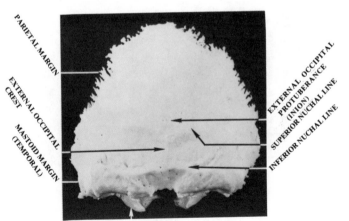

EXTERNAL VIEW

FIGURE 3-12
SPHENOID BONE

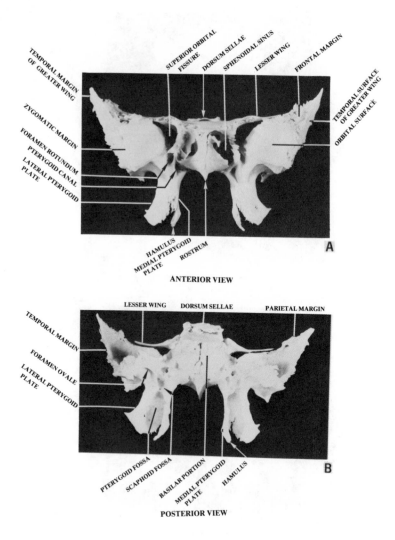

ANTERIOR VIEW

POSTERIOR VIEW

FIGURE 3-13
ETHMOID BONE

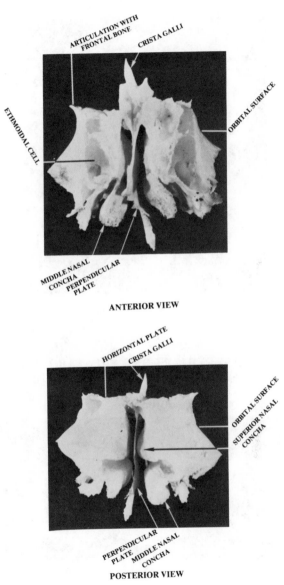

ARTICULATION WITH FRONTAL BONE

CRISTA GALLI

ORBITAL SURFACE

ETHMOIDAL CELL

MIDDLE NASAL CONCHA

PERPENDICULAR PLATE

ANTERIOR VIEW

HORIZONTAL PLATE

CRISTA GALLI

ORBITAL SURFACE

SUPERIOR NASAL CONCHA

PERPENDICULAR PLATE

MIDDLE NASAL CONCHA

POSTERIOR VIEW

FIGURE 3-14
ETHMOID BONE & INFERIOR NASAL CONCHA

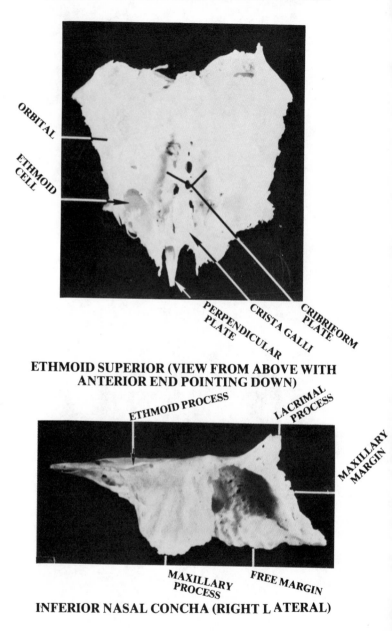

ORBITAL

ETHMOID CELL

PERPENDICULAR PLATE

CRISTA GALLI

CRIBRIFORM PLATE

ETHMOID SUPERIOR (VIEW FROM ABOVE WITH ANTERIOR END POINTING DOWN)

ETHMOID PROCESS

LACRIMAL PROCESS

MAXILLARY MARGIN

MAXILLARY PROCESS

FREE MARGIN

INFERIOR NASAL CONCHA (RIGHT L ATERAL)

FIGURE 3-14 (Continued)
ETHMOID BONE & INFERIOR NASAL CONCHA

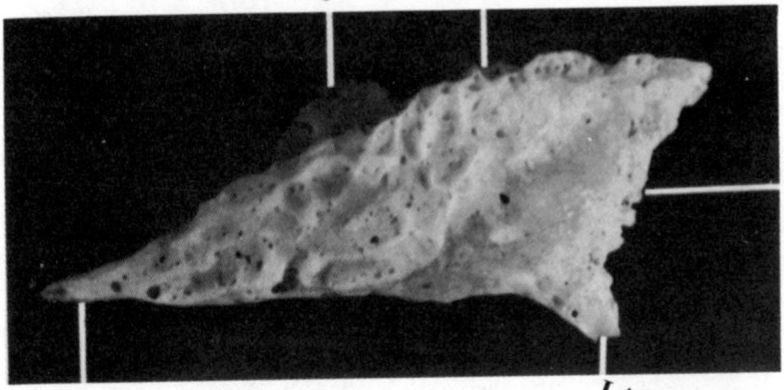

INFERIOR NASAL CONCHA (RIGHT MEDIAL)

NOTE: Approximate relative sizes of adult ethmoid and inferior nasal concha bones are not apparent in Figure 3-14. Sizes of typical specimens are:

Ethmoid
  Height - 3⅔ cm
  Width - Apex - 2 cm
       Broadest width, just above base - 3½ cm

Inferior Nasal Concha
  Height - 3½ cm (longest axis)
  Width - across center of bone - ⅓ cm

individuals. Controversially, the variability may account for some differences in voice quality. The sinuses can be demonstrated best in a skull whose outer and inner tables have been carefully separated. Such skulls are commercially available, although at high cost.

The sphenoid sinus is in the body of the sphenoid bone anterior and inferior to the sella turcica. The ethmoid cells are posterior to the orbital plates of the ethmoid bone and communicate with the area under the superior nasal conchae. The frontal sinuses are large inconstant chambers in the frontal bone. The maxillary sinus fills the body of the maxilla on each side.

FIGURE 3-15
LACRIMAL, NASAL AND VOMER BONES

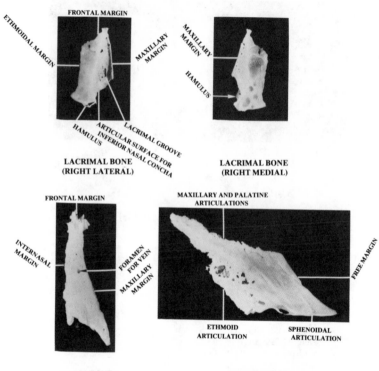

LACRIMAL BONE
(RIGHT LATERAL)

LACRIMAL BONE
(RIGHT MEDIAL)

NASAL BONE
(LEFT ANTERIOR)

VOMER BONE
(LATERAL)

The nasal septum divides the nasal passage into two chambers. The septum is composed of cartilages anteriorly, the perpendicular plate of the ethmoid posteriorly and superiorly, and the vomer bone posteriorly and inferiorly.

The openings of the nasal passages into the pharynx are the choanae narium. Each choana is formed by the palatine bone, medial

FIGURE 3-16
ZYGOMATIC BONE

FRONTAL PROCESS (MARGIN)

ZYGOMATICOFACIAL FORAMEN

INFRAORBITAL MARGIN

MAXILLARY MARGIN

TEMPORAL PROCESS (MARGIN)

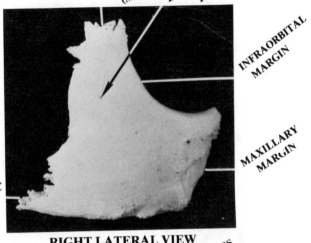

RIGHT LATERAL VIEW

ORBITAL SURFACE

FRONTAL PROCESS (MARGIN)

ZYGOMATICO-ORBITAL FORAMEN

MAXILLARY MARGIN

TEMPORAL PROCESS (MARGIN)

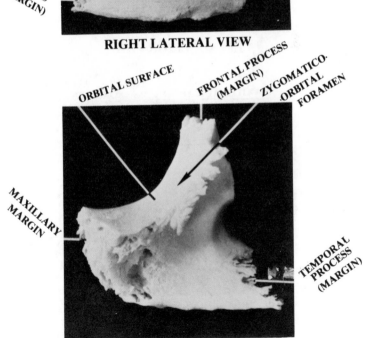

LEFT LATERAL VIEW

FIGURE 3-17
PALATINE BONE

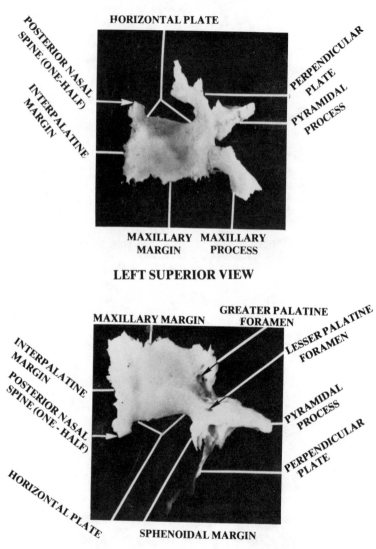

LEFT SUPERIOR VIEW

LEFT INFERIOR VIEW

FIGURE 3-17 (Continued)
PALATINE BONE

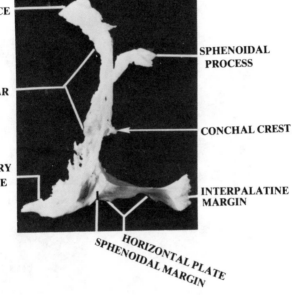

ORBITAL SURFACE

SPHENOIDAL PROCESS

PERPENDICULAR PLATE

CONCHAL CREST

MAXILLARY SURFACE

INTERPALATINE MARGIN

HORIZONTAL PLATE

SPHENOIDAL MARGIN

LEFT POSTERIOR VIEW

pterygoid plate, and vomer. The nasal passages open to the outside through the anterior nares.

Disarticulated Bones

If time permits, examine in detail various disarticulated bones (all available commercially). The salient features of such bones are illustrated in this text.

FIGURE 3-18
MAXILLARY BONE

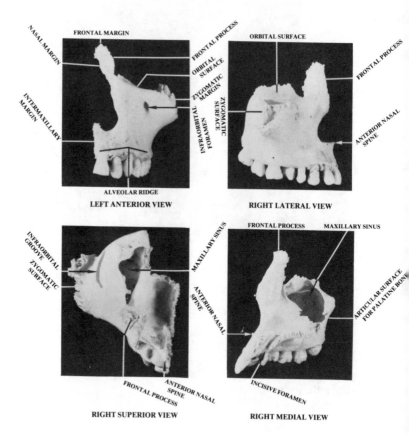

LEFT ANTERIOR VIEW

RIGHT LATERAL VIEW

RIGHT SUPERIOR VIEW

RIGHT MEDIAL VIEW

FIGURE 3-19
HYOID BONE

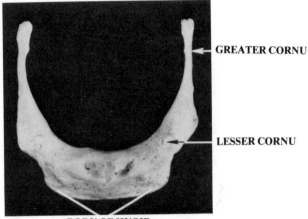

GREATER CORNU

LESSER CORNU

BODY OF HYOID

SUPERIOR VIEW

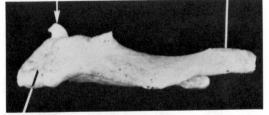

LESSER CORNU

GREATER CORNU

BODY OF HYOID

LATERAL VIEW

FIGURE 3-20
MANDIBLE

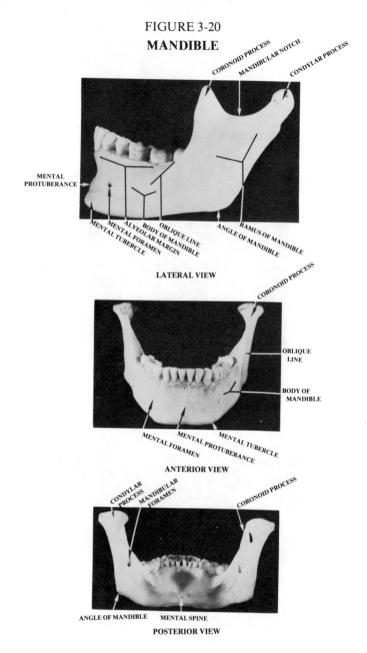

LATERAL VIEW

ANTERIOR VIEW

POSTERIOR VIEW

EXERCISE 4

FACIAL, MANDIBULAR AND EXTRINSIC LARYNGEAL MUSCLES IN MAN

OBJECTIVES

There are hundreds of muscles in the human body. Certain representative groups which are of importance in the activities of speech have been selected for study.

The muscles of facial expression are intimately involved in communication, a term which embraces non-verbal as well as verbal activities. The student should appreciate the relationship of the geographic positions of the facial muscles to their functioning.

The movements of the mandible are related to articulation as well as to chewing and the mandibular muscles should be studied with particular regard to articulation of sounds.

The muscles that elevate and depress the larynx are essential to the process of phonation and efforts should be made to identify their positions, relationships and actions. The intrinsic laryngeal muscles are not considered in the present Exercise.

TIME REQUIRED

One laboratory period - two hours

MATERIALS

Models and charts, emphasizing muscle attachments on the face, mandible, neck and larynx

Human skeletons and isolated skulls

Reference texts in human anatomy

Access if possible to prosected human cadavers

Preserved cats

DESCRIPTION

It is difficult to comprehend function if the muscles examined are not in action. This same difficulty is apparent in studying human skeletons, charts, models and even well illustrated texts, Nevertheless, a variety of visual aids should be available so that muscles of relevance can be identified and their actions made clear. It is feasible to study speech muscles in action through electromyography, but recording systems are expensive and evaluations require sophisticated knowledge and experience. Some basic aspects of the EMG will be considered later in this text.

The standard methods of physical diagnosis help understand muscle function. These methods include inspection and palpation to outline muscles and to test their status in living action. Weakness and/or atrophy are the common clinical parameters evaluated. The necessity for clinical experience precludes utilizing the detailed procedures, although a few general observations are considered in this Exercise.

PROCEDURE

Mimetic and Other Facial Musculature

The orbicularis oculi is the principal muscle encircling the eye, acting more as a sphincter than as a muscle of expression. The palpebral portion covering the eyelids closes the lids, as in blinking. The orbital part forms the larger mass, palpated as an ellipse surrounding the orbit. The contraction of this circumferential mass closes the eyes. Test these functions in a subject.

Muscles such as the nasalis, procerus, occipitofrontalis, auricularis, and others are involved in movements of the scalp and upper face. Test these movements in a subject.

The muscles around the lips, arising in the central or lower facial region include the following:

Levator labii superioris	Depressor labii inferioris
Levator labii superioris alaeque nasi	Depressor anguli oris
Levator anguli oris	Mentalis
Zygomaticus minor	Orbicularis oris
Zygomaticus major	Buccinator
Risorius	

Acting in groups, the central and lower muscles provide a wide range of movements of the lips and cheeks for speech and for nonveroal, expressive communication.

FIGURE 4-1
DEEP FACIAL MUSCLES

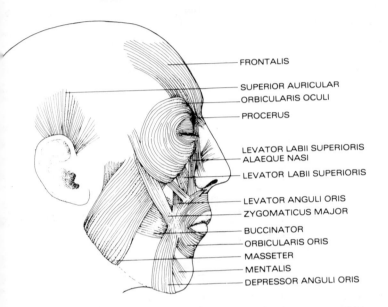

FRONTALIS

SUPERIOR AURICULAR
ORBICULARIS OCULI

PROCERUS

LEVATOR LABII SUPERIORIS
ALAEQUE NASI

LEVATOR LABII SUPERIORIS

LEVATOR ANGULI ORIS
ZYGOMATICUS MAJOR

BUCCINATOR
ORBICULARIS ORIS

MASSETER

MENTALIS
DEPRESSOR ANGULI ORIS

If possible, have the muscles demonstrated in the prosected human cadaver. Study the activity of these muscles by inspection during forced facial expressions among laboratory partners.

Line drawings of predominating facial features suggesting basic expressions can be made available. Complete each drawing by adding in outline the muscles most actively involved. Use charts and head models adjunctively to fulfill the task.

Muscles of the Mandible

The muscles that depress the mandible will be considered under the suprahyoid group. The following are mainly elevators. Note the actions of the temporalis and masseter muscles by inspection and palpation during chewing. Draw the mandible in outline and sketch in all other muscles of this bone. Using a skull and a mandible, cut out models of the muscles and place them by tape into their positions of origin and insertion. Refer to Exercise 3 for views of the bony mandible.

The temporalis is a flat muscle originating from the temporal fossa on the parietal, temporal and frontal bones. It inserts into the coronoid process of the mandible and the anterior border of the ramus of the mandible. It elevates the mandible.

FIGURE 4-2
CHEWING MUSCLES

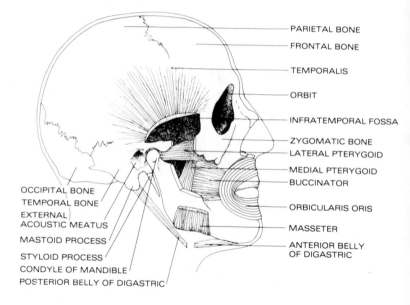

The masseter is a powerful muscle which elevates the mandible. It arises from two heads on the zygomatic arch and it inserts on the mandible at its angle and along the postero-lateral aspect of its ramus.

The medial pterygoid roughly parallels the masseter, but it travels on the inside of the ramus of the mandible. The muscle originates mainly from the lateral pterygoid plate of the sphenoid bone. Together, the masseter and the medial pterygoid form a sling suspending the angle of the mandible. Both muscles elevate the mandible.

The lateral pterygoid muscle opposes the action of the other muscles of mastication by depressing the mandible. Originating from the great wing of the sphenoid and the lateral pterygoid plate, the fibers run dorsally to attach to the condyle of the mandible. The muscle also protrudes the mandible and moves it from side to side.

Muscles that Elevate the Hyoid Bone and the Larynx

This group comprises the suprahyoid muscles. Acting from below they can depress the mandible.

Student groups can best study the laryngeal elevators (and the depressors) in prosected human cadavers or even in preserved cats. Students are also referred to Exercise 17 on electromyography.

FIGURE 4-3
ELEVATORS AND DEPRESSORS OF THE LARYNX
(SCHEMATIC)

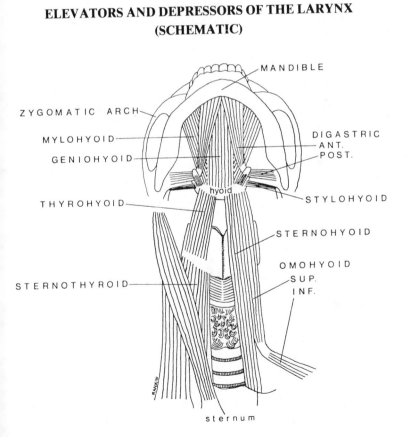

The following reconstruction can be prepared. Draw a diagrammatic figure containing mandible, tongue, temporal bone, sternum, scapulae, pharynx, larynx and hyoid bone. With colored crayons, show the muscles connecting these structures to the hyoid bone. Consider in sketches the changed position of the hyoid as the various muscles described below go into action.

The digastric muscle has a posterior belly originating in the mastoid notch of the temporal bone and an anterior belly originating from the lower aspect of the mandible. The two bellies unite in a tendon which is tied down to the hyoid bone.

The anterior belly raises and draws forward the hyoid bone. The posterior belly raises and draws back the hyoid bone. The muscle acting from the hyoid can depress the mandible.

The stylohyoid muscle originates in the styloid process of the temporal bone and passes down and forward to the hyoid bone. It draws the hyoid up and back.

The mylohyoid muscle forms the floor of the mouth. The muscle on each side originates from the mylohyoid line on the medial aspect of the mandible and the anterior and middle fibers insert into a central raphe which extends from the mandibular symphysis to the hyoid bone. The posterior fibers travel centrally and downward to the hyoid. The muscle elevates both the tongue and the hyoid bone. In reverse, it depresses the mandible.

The geniohyoid muscle is deep to the mylohyoid. Originating on the mental spines behind the mandibular symphysis, the geniohyoids travel on either side of the midline down and back to the hyoid bone. They draw the hyoid and tongue forward or, in reverse, they depress the mandible.

Muscles that Depress the Larynx

These are the infrahyoid muscles. If the pharynx and larynx have been elevated, as in swallowing, the infrahyoid muscles lower the hyoid bone and the larynx. These muscles are visualized clearly in the human cadaver or preserved cat. Draw the larynx and trachea in outline and sketch in these muscles.

The omohyoid muscle consists of two bellies coming together at a central tendon. Originating at the upper border of the scapula or from the ligament that crosses the scapular notch, the inferior belly travels

FIGURE 4-4
EXTRINSIC MUSCLES OF LARYNX

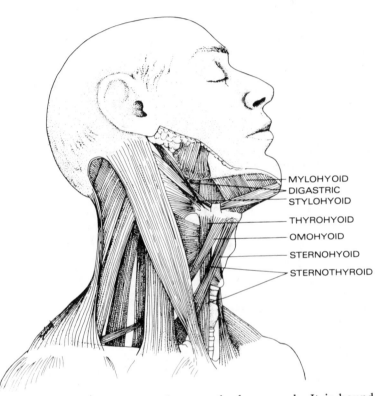

MYLOHYOID
DIGASTRIC
STYLOHYOID

THYROHYOID

OMOHYOID

STERNOHYOID

STERNOTHYROID

forward and somewhat upward across the lower neck. It is bound down to the clavicle but emerges and travels behind the sternocleidomastoid muscle where it forms a tendon which terminates by union with the superior belly. The latter goes almost vertically upward, parallel with the outer edge of the sternohyoid, and inserts into the lower aspect of the hyoid bone body. The muscle depresses the hyoid bone.

The thyrohyoid muscle looks as though it continued the sternothyroid muscle upward. Its origin is from an oblique line on the right and left laminae of the thyroid cartilage. Its insertion is on the greater cornua of the hyoid bone. It can depress the hyoid, although it can elevate the thyroid cartilage.

The sternothyroid muscle originates from the manubrium of the sternum and the first costal cartilage and it inserts on each side into the thyroid cartilage lamina. It depresses the thyroid cartilage.

The sternohyoid muscle originates in the sternal manubrium, medial clavicle, and sternoclavicular ligament. It travels upwards, both members lying side by side from the middle of their course, and it inserts into the lower aspect of the body of the hyoid bone. It depresses this bone.

NOTE: The student can profit by making schematic diagrams showing probable direction (and extent) of movement of structures because of muscle contraction. Such diagrams are effective in suggesting that muscles can act from more than one source and in coordination. This procedure is a useful adjunct to the study of diagrams that emphasize contraction of any single muscle.

REFERENCES

Exercise 1

DiFiore, M.S.H. **Atlas of Human Histology.** 4th ed. Philadelphia: Lea and Febiger, 1974.

Ham, A. W. and Cormack, D. H. **Histology.** 8th Ed. Philadelphia: J.B. Lippincott Company, 1979.

Nicolosi, L., Harryman, E. and Kresheck, J. **Terminology of Communication Disorders.** Baltimore: Williams and Wilkins, 1978.

Porter, K. and Bonneville, M. **Fine Structure of Cells and Tissues.** Philadelphia: Lea and Febiger, 1973.

Robbins, S. D. **A Dicitonary of Speech Pathology and Therapy.** 2nd ed. Cambridge, Mass.: Sci-Art Publishers, 1963.

Exercises 2 & 3

Anderson, J. E. **Grant's Atlas of Anatomy.** 7th ed. Baltimore: Williams and Wilkins Company, 1978.

Langman, J. and Woerdeman, M. **Atlas of Medical Anatomy.** Philadelphia: W. B. Saunders Company, 1977.

McMinn, R. M. H. and Hutchings, R.T. **Color Atlas of Human Anatomy.** Chicago: Year Book Medical Publishers, 1977.

Spalteholz, W. and Spanner, R. **Atlas of Human Anatomy.** 16th ed. Philadelphia: F.A. Davis Company, 1967.

Warwick, R. and Williams, P. L. **Gray's Anatomy.** 36th ed. Philadephia: W. B. Saunders Company, 1980.

Exercise 4

Basmajian, J.V. **Muscles Alive.** 3rd ed. Baltimore: The Williams and Wilkins Company, 1974.

Brunnstrom, S. and Dickinson, R. **Clinical Kinesiology.** 3rd ed. Phildelphia: F. A. Davis Company, 1972.

Warwick, R. and Williams, P. L. **Gray's Anatomy.** 6th ed. Philadelphia: W. B. Saunders Company, 1980.

CHAPTER II

Neuroanatomy and Neurophysiology

EXERCISE 5

ANATOMY OF THE SHEEP BRAIN

OBJECTIVES

The student should be able to identify the general structures and subdivisions of the sheep brain, its cranial nerves, ventricles, major commissures, and meninges. This is an introduction to understanding the landmarks of the more anatomically complex human brain which is the subject matter of Exercise 6. Sheep brains are readily available commercially and they are the classical type forms for the introductory student. The instructor should emphasize that there are undefined functional differences between the animal and the human brain.

TIME REQUIRED

One laboratory period - two hours

MATERIALS

Whole and sagittally-sectioned, preserved sheep brains

Pans, pointers, forceps, disposable gloves

DESCRIPTION AND PROCEDURE

I. Whole Isolated Brain

Norma Verticalis

This is the dorsal (superior) view, looking down from above (Figure 5-1). The cerebral hemispheres, the cerebellum, and the spinal cord are all visible in this view. If the cerebral hemispheres are lifted in front, the olfactory bulbs can be seen. Note that the surface of the cerebral hemispheres is convoluted into hills called gyri and valleys called sulci.

The term fissure refers to a deep groove and the term sulcus refers to a shallow groove. Observe that there are many fissures seen in surface views. Find the median longitudinal fissure which is a midsagittal cut that divides the two cerebral hemispheres. A median dorsal fissure partially divides the spinal cord along its length. A transverse cerebral fissure marks the cerebrum off from the cerebellum.

In the space between the cerebrum and cerebellum, locate the structures lying in the dorsal aspect of the midbrain. In this space there are prominent bodies called the corpora quadrigemina. These bodies are deep and the student needs to separate the cerebrum and cerebellum to visualize them. They are thus not labelled in Figure 5-1

Observe the lateral aspects of the spinal cord while the specimen is viewed in dorsal aspect. Note the roots of the spinal nerves emerging from the cord. These roots are to be examined in more detail later.

Norma Basalis

This is the ventral view of the brain (Figure 5-2). Students will find this to be the best view for studying the cranial nerves.

Identify the following structures with the help of Figure 5-2. The large olfactory bulbs and olfactory tracts are prominent at

FIGURE 5-1
NORMA VERTICALIS OF THE SHEEP BRAIN

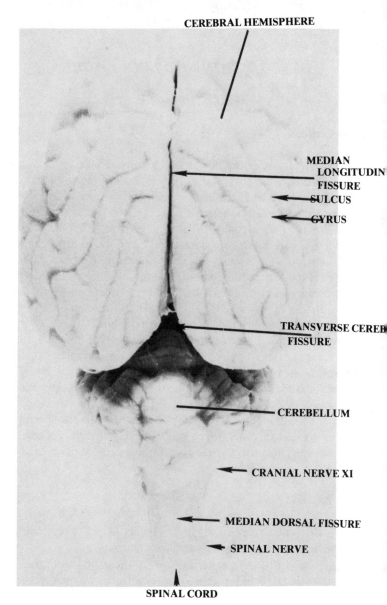

CEREBRAL HEMISPHERE

MEDIAN LONGITUDIN FISSURE

SULCUS

GYRUS

TRANSVERSE CEREB FISSURE

CEREBELLUM

CRANIAL NERVE XI

MEDIAN DORSAL FISSURE

SPINAL NERVE

SPINAL CORD

FIGURE 5-2
NORMA BASALIS OF THE SHEEP BRAIN

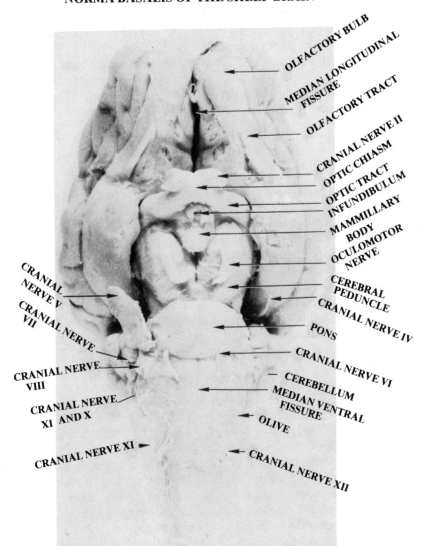

OLFACTORY BULB

MEDIAN LONGITUDINAL FISSURE

OLFACTORY TRACT

CRANIAL NERVE II

OPTIC CHIASM

OPTIC TRACT

INFUNDIBULUM

MAMMILLARY BODY

OCULOMOTOR NERVE

CEREBRAL PEDUNCLE

CRANIAL NERVE IV

PONS

CRANIAL NERVE VI

CEREBELLUM

MEDIAN VENTRAL FISSURE

OLIVE

CRANIAL NERVE XII

CRANIAL NERVE V

CRANIAL NERVE VII

CRANIAL NERVE VIII

CRANIAL NERVE XI AND X

CRANIAL NERVE XI

the most cranial aspect. The median longitudinal fissure separates the paired bulbs. Moving caudally, find the optic chiasm in the ventral midline. The optic tracts lead to the x-shaped chiasm, and the optic nerves (cranial nerve II) travel distally on the right and left to innervate the eyes. Caudal to the chiasm, the infundibulum (tube-like stalk of the pituitary gland) is attached.

A rounded eminence, the mammillary body, rises caudal to the attachment of the infundibulum. The oculomotor nerve (cranial nerve III) arises laterally and caudally to the mammillary body just medial to the cerebral peduncles.

Embryology

A bit of embryological terminology may serve to give the student an appreciation of the structures he is observing. The brain develops first as structures around three cavities (vesicles) in linear cranio-caudal sequence. The vesicles and their walls form the forebrain, midbrain and hindbrain, or prosencephalon, mesencephalon and rhombencephalon, respectively. The prosencephalon divides to a telencephalon cranially and a diencephalon caudally.

The telencephalon consists of the cerebral hemispheres and the olfactory bulbs and it comprises the bulk of the brain. The diencephalon is made up of the thalamus, epithalamus, metathalamus, and hypothalamus. The hypothalamus gives rise to the infundibulum and optic tracts.

The mesencephalon is represented in basal aspect by the cerebral peduncles. The peduncles appear as two thick stalks joined in the middle, linking the forebrain and the midbrain. The trochlear nerve (cranial nerve IV) arises on either side of the mesencephalon and is just inferior to the corpora quadrigemina.

The rhombencephalon is divided into a metencephalon cranially and a myelencephalon caudally. In the ventral (basal) view, a prominent body called the pons occupies the metencephalon. The myelencephalon develops to the medulla oblongata. A median ventral fissure divides the medulla to right and left halves.

Turning the specimen to the norma verticalis (dorsal view) to complete the embryological description, the cranial aspect of the dorsal rhombencephalon, or metencephalon, becomes the cerebellum. The caudal aspect is the dorsal myelecephalon, or medulla oblongata.

Cranial Nerves

These are best visualized in ventral view (norma basalis) where their roots leave the brain. The student should isolate and identify all pairs of nerves not seen previously.

The trigeminal nerve (V cranial) arises from the dorso-lateral aspect of the pons. The trigeminal is the largest of the cranial nerves. Emerging between the pons and the medulla, observe the abducent nerve (VI cranial). Cranial nerves VII and VIII, the facial and acoustic nerves, can be seen leaving the hindbrain dorsal to the olive near the trigeminal nerve. From a groove between the olive and the caudal cerebellar peduncle, observe the roots of the glossopharyngeal and vagus nerves (IX and X cranials). More medially and toward the caudal limit of the medulla, several rootlets coalesce to constitute the hypoglossal (XII cranial) nerve. The accessory nerve (XI cranial) arises from several rootlets in a line with the vagus which unite to form a nerve trunk on the lateral aspect of the medulla and cord.

Norma Lateralis

This is the lateral view of the brain. The student should study the structures therein, following this text and referring to Figure 5-3.

Note that a single cerebral hemisphere dominates this view. In the dorsal hindbrain observe the cerebellar hemisphere. Below the cerebellum observe the medulla oblongata leading caudally into the spinal cord. Cranial to the medulla, note the pons which protrudes slightly ventrally.

Immediately cranial to the pons, the large cerebral peduncles extend to the forebrain. Pull the cerebrum down to reveal the recessed dorsal corpora quadrigemina, which consist of the four colliculi (two cranial and two caudal). The pineal body is cranial to the colliculi. It is not visible in surface view.

The large olfactory tract and bulb are visible. The optic chiasm can be seen hanging from the middle of the forebrain. Follow this cranially to see the pituitary gland which is supported by a stalk, the infundibulum.

Several cranial nerves are visible in the lateral view. Observe the spinal accessory nerve (XI) running parallel and in juxtaposition to the cord. Several roots from the most caudal and ventral aspects of the

FIGURE 5-3
NORMA LATERALIS OF THE SHEEP BRAIN

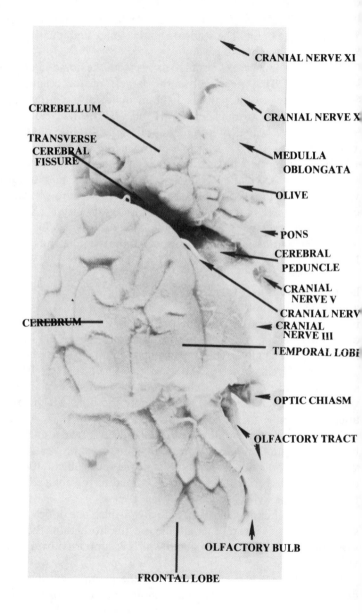

CRANIAL NERVE XI

CRANIAL NERVE X

CEREBELLUM

TRANSVERSE
CEREBRAL
FISSURE

MEDULLA
OBLONGATA

OLIVE

PONS

CEREBRAL
PEDUNCLE

CRANIAL
NERVE V

CRANIAL NERV

CRANIAL
NERVE III

CEREBRUM

TEMPORAL LOBE

OPTIC CHIASM

OLFACTORY TRACT

OLFACTORY BULB

FRONTAL LOBE

medulla oblongata give rise to the hypoglossal nerve (XII). An oblong, raised structure, the olive, protrudes just cranial to the hypoglossal nerve. Cranial to the olive a number of nerve roots are visible which combine to form the glossopharyngeal (IX) and the vagus (X) nerves. The large bundle of roots forming the trigeminal nerve (V) is apparent near the pons. Ventral and somewhat caudal to the trigeminal, the facial nerve (VII) and acoustic nerve (VIH) are seen.

II. Mid-Sagittal Section Of The Brain

The student is to refer to Figure 5-4. The mid-sagittal view allows visualization of the internal canal system through which the cerebrospinal fluid flows. The canal system enlarges to a set of four ventricles in specific parts of the internal brain.

There is a pair of lateral ventricles within each cerebral hemisphere. Note the single member of the pair in your cut specimen.

A thick band, the corpus callosum plus the fornix, surrounds the lateral ventricle. These white fibers, which connect the hemispheres, are commissures. The corpus callosum is the dorsal band. The fornix is the diagonal strip running from the caudal end of the corpus callosum to the diencephalon. What are the functions of these commissures?

The lateral ventricles are closed and separated by a membrane, the septum pellucidum. The lateral ventricles communicate with the third ventricle lying directly caudal to the fornix. A canal, the cerebral aqueduct, passes caudally above the cerebral peduncles to the base of the cerebellum. The fourth ventricle is in the hindbrain and it is continuous caudally with the central canal of the spinal cord. The fourth ventricle is located between the stalks, or peduncles, which connect the dorsally located cerebellum to other parts of the brain. Probe the ventricles, tracing their paths through the brain.

Locate the cranial, middle and caudal cerebellar peduncles on each side. Trace them dorsally to the cerebellum. Observe the internal structure of the cerebellum which resembles a "tree of life," or arbor vitae.

Identify the corpora quadrigemina and the pineal body which are dorsal and cranial to the cerebellum.

FIGURE 5-4
MIDSAGITTAL SECTION OF THE SHEEP BRAIN

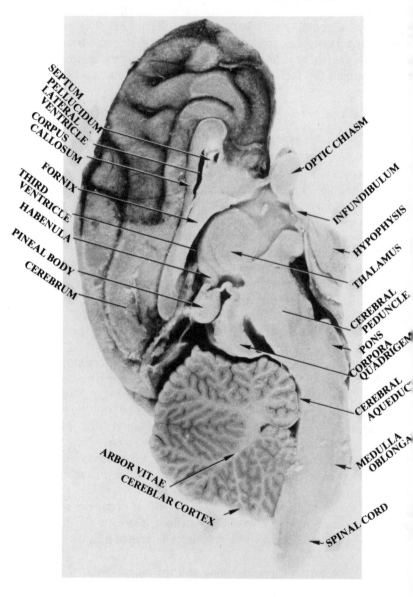

SEPTUM PELLUCIDUM
LATERAL VENTRICLE
CORPUS CALLOSUM
FORNIX
THIRD VENTRICLE
HABENULA
PINEAL BODY
CEREBRUM
ARBOR VITAE
CEREBLAR CORTEX

OPTIC CHIASM
INFUNDIBULUM
HYPOPHYSIS
THALAMUS
CEREBRAL PEDUNCLE
PONS
CORPORA QUADRIGEN
CEREBRAL AQUEDUC
MEDULLA OBLONGA
SPINAL CORD

In the diencephalon, observe the infundibulum, mammillary body and optic tracts along the ventral border of the cut brain. Dorsal to these structures, locate the hypothalamus. At the end of the peduncles and dorsal to the hypothalamus, find the thalamus. Caudal to the upper part of the fornix, the habenula and the pineal body form the epithalamus.

EXERCISE 6

ANATOMY OF THE HUMAN BRAIN

OBJECTIVES

The student should identify the prominent structural features of the isolated, preserved human brain. This can provide an anatomic basis for understanding the neural regulation of speech and the possible specialization of functions with relation to areas of the brain.

TIME REQUIRED

Two laboratory periods - four hours

MATERIALS

Isolated whole human brains; also specimens which are cut both midsagittally and coronally

Brain charts, models and anatomic atlases
Pans, forceps, probes

Note: Preserved wet specimens of human brains can be made available by arrangement with the medical departments of anatomy. With careful handling they can be kept for several years. Excellent "plastomounts" and preserved specimens of the human brain can also be purchased (Carolina Biological Supply Co., Burlington, N.C. 27215) by the instructional department.

DESCRIPTION AND PROCEDURE

Follow the descriptions herein. One student reads the outline while others locate the structures. Refer to the four figures and their keys. Have charts and atlases available.

I. General Observations

Observe that the brain is covered by meninges. The dura mater is the outermost, tough fibrous covering. Inside the dura a net-like film, the arachnoid membrane, surrounds the brain. The third, or innermost layer called the pia mater, covers the brain intimately. Locate these meninges, then strip off the two outer membranes to visualize the brain structures, proper.

Turn your attention to whatever arteries remain on the isolated brain. There are four great arteries which run up the neck to the brain. These are the paired internal carotids ventrally and the paired vertebral arteries dorsally. The carotid arteries enter the cranium through the carotid canals. The vertebral arteries enter through the foramen magnum. The vertebral arteries unite to form the basilar artery which is ventral to the pons. The basilar artery branches into right and left posterior cerebral arteries. Each carotid artery bifurcates to form the anterior cerebral artery and middle cerebral artery. Communicating branches connect the two anterior cerebral arteries as they branch from the carotids and connect the middle cerebral artery to the posterior cerebral artery on both sides. The interconnections form the circle of Willis on the base of the brain. The circle in turn sends blood vessels to the various regions of the brain.

Review the embryology described in Exercise 5 and recall that the brain develops first as three vesicles. The forebrain (prosencephalon) specializes to such major structures as the cerebral hemispheres, thalami, epithalami, subthalami, and hypothalami. The midbrain (mesencephalon) develops such important structures as the cerebral peduncles and corpora quadrigemina. The hindbrain (rhombencephalon) develops the cerebellum, pons, and medulla.

II. Geographic Regions of the Brain

Use atlases and the accompanying figures to find all structures from this point on. Keep repositioning the brain as needed.

Telencephalon

This is the anterior (cranial; cephalic; rostral) part of the forebrain (prosencephalon). The cerebral hemispheres develop from it and grow dorsally over most of the other structures, thus obscuring them (Figures 6-1 through 6-4). Note in the dorsal view (Figure 6-2) the separation of the cerebrum to right and left hemisphere by the longitudinal cerebral fissure. Note the gyri and sulci which greatly increase the surface area in the cerebral hemispheres. Observe the surface division to four lobes, resulting from the great fissures of Sylvius and Rolando. The lobes are not units of function, but rather multifunctional.

Lift the cerebrum dorsally and observe the olfactory bulbs beneath the frontal lobes and also the olfactory tracts that lead into the bulbs. These structures transmit olfactory impulses from nasal receptors to the "smell" brain (rhinencephalon).

Diencephalon

This is the caudal part of the forebrain (prosencephalon). The diencephalon is composed of the paired bodies of the thalamus, and epithalamus, subthalamus and hypothalamus.

The diencephalon encloses the third ventricle. This space plus the fourth ventricle, two lateral ventricles in the cerebral hemispheres, and the passages which connect all the ventricles make up the ventricular system. These chambers and passages provide a route for the cerebrospinal fluid to bathe the brain. The spaces are confluent with the subarachnoid space around the brain and the spinal cord. The foramen of Monro connects the lateral ventricles to the third ventricle. The cerebral aqueduct is the passage between the third and fourth ventricles. The ventricles can be visualized best in midsagittal section of the brain (Figure 6-3).

The thalami are large, paired ovoid masses on the right and left

FIGURE 6-1
NORMA LATERALIS OF THE HUMAN BRAIN

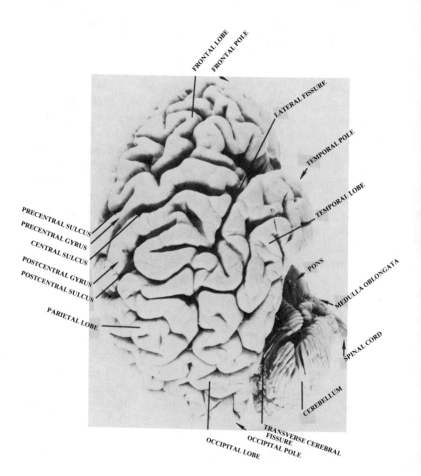

sides of the third ventricle. The thalamus can be seen only in sagittal section (Figure 6-3). Each thalamus consists chiefly of gray substance which is divided to many nuclei.

The epithalamus occupies the caudal part of the roof of the diencephalon. The term epithalamus includes the unpaired pineal body, paired habenula (trigonum habenulae) and the posterior commissure.

FIGURE 6-2

NORMA VERTICALIS OF THE HUMAN BRAIN

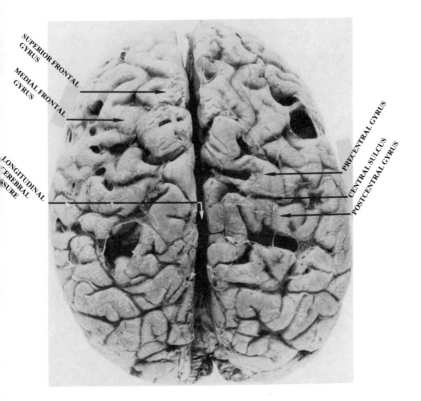

The pineal body is a pea-sized structure lying above the superior colliculi. A stalk-like projection composed of the posterior commissure and the habenula supports the pineal body. The posterior commissure is a band of white fibers. Part of the band connects the paired superior colliculi.

The subthalamus (ventral thalamus) is wedged in between the cerebral peduncle and the mammillary area. The hypothalamus is cranial and medial to it. The subthalamus contains the nucleus subthalamicus and also fiber masses called the fields of Forel.

FIGURE 6-3
MIDSAGITTAL SECTION OF THE HUMAN BRAIN

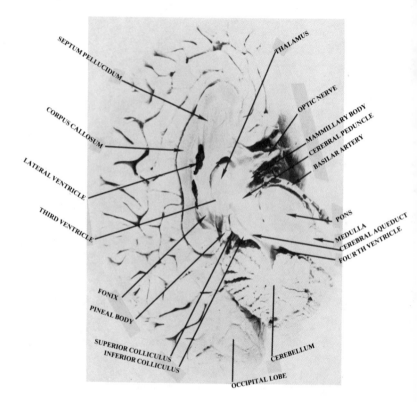

The hypothalamus is an extremely important diencephalic structure and is divided to many parts, e.g. mammillary bodies, tuber cinereum, pituitary gland, infundibulum. Refer to Figure 6-4 (norma basalis) and Figure 6-3 (midsagittal section). The hypothalamus extends from the optic chiasm (chiasma) in front through the mammillary bodies behind and it forms the floor and cephalic part of the wall of the third ventricle. Its functions are numerous and the student is referred to standard textbooks of human physiology.

The optic chiasm can be seen in the basal view in the floor of the

FIGURE 6-4
NORMA BASALIS OF THE HUMAN BRAIN

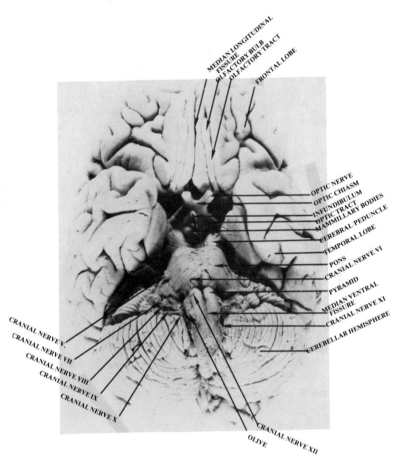

diencephalon, appearing as a single, prominent X-shaped configuration (Figure 6-4). It contains fibers of the right and left optic nerves passing from the retina of the eyes toward the brain.

The infundibulum, or single stalk from the hypothalamus to the pituitary gland (hypophysis), is seen in the basal view to be just above (dorsal) to the chiasm.

The mammillary bodies are also dorsal to the optic chiasm (Figure 6-3). These bodies are two small, rounded protuberances. Observe in basal view the paired oculomotor (third cranial) nerves which exit from the brain just behind the mammillary bodies.

Study the midsagittally sectioned brain. Locate the anterior commissure, the fornix, the corpus callosum, the lateral ventricles, the septum pellucidum, and the lamina terminalis.

The corpus callosum is a large C-shaped band of white fibers that helps connect the right and left cerebral hemispheres. Such horizontal interconnecting bands are called commissures. They also include the fornix and the anterior commissure.

The anterior commissure is above the optic chiasm and appears as an oval connection between the cerebral hemispheres which have been separated. The commissure is a bundle of white fibers which decussate (cross the midline). Most of these fibers connect the amygdalae and pyriform areas which are parts of the "smell" brain (rhinencephalon). Some travel to the temporal cortex.

The fornix is a paired band of fibers lying close to the median plane. The band fuses in its middle region and travels ventrally to the corpus callosum over the thalamus. At the highest part of its C-shaped arch, the body of the fornix is dorsal to the roof of the third ventricle and it is just ventral to the septum pellucidum.

The septum pellucidum is between the corpus callosum and fornix and it has no commissural fibers. The septum covers the opening into the lateral ventricle on each side. The paired lateral ventricles must then empty their cerebrospinal fluid into the central foramen of Monro for the fluid to travel more caudally into the single third ventricle. The septum pellucidum thus acts as a narrow partition between the paired lateral ventricles.

The lateral ventricles are separated within the cerebral hemispheres. The roof of each is the ventral surface of the corpus callosum. The medial boundary of each is the septum pellucidum. The floor has a number of bodies, including the lateral aspect of the fornix, thalamus. caudate nucleus, stria and vena terminalis, and choroid plexus. These bodies need not be differentiated here.

The lamina terminalis may be seen as a thin, ridge-like structure which extends from the anterior commissure toward the optic chiasm.

Midbrain (Mesencephalon)

The midbrain is a short segment connecting the forebrain with the cerebellum and the pons. Its dorsal aspect, or tectum, contains the corpora quadrigemina. Its ventral aspect contains the cerebral peduncles.

The peduncles can be seen as two ridges which diverge as they travel toward the cerebral hemispheres. The space formed between the ridges is the interpeduncular fossa whose floor is the posterior perforated substance.

The corpora quadrigemina (colliculi) are seen as two pairs of rounded lobes in the dorsal aspect of the midbrain (Figure 6-3). The rostral pair are superior colliculi and the caudal pair are the inferior colliculi. The trochlear (IV) nerves emerge just caudal to each inferior colliculus.

There is a transitional area between the superior colliculi and the thalamus which is called the pretectal region. It accepts fibers from the optic tract and sends fibers to the Edinger-Westphal nucleus of the oculomotor nerve, thus providing reflex eyeball responses to retinal impulses.

Hindbrain (Rhombencephalon)

The hindbrain plus the midbrain constitutes the brainstem. Its rostral aspect (metencephalon) contains the cerebellum dorsally and the pons ventrally. Its caudal aspect (myelencephalon) contains the medulla oblongata both dorsally and ventrally.

The fourth ventricle is the spinal fluid bearing cavity in the hindbrain. It opens rostrally into the cerebral aqueduct and caudally into the central canal of the medulla. Its roof contains a network of blood vessels called a choroid plexus. The plexus allows transudation of ventricular spinal fluid into the subarachnoid space within the meninges around this region. The floor, or ventral wall of the fourth ventricle, is occupied by the rhomboid fossa. This is produced by the dorsal surface of the pons and of the cranial part of the medulla.

Locate the pons in basal and midsagittal views (Figures 6-3 and 6-4). The pons is a prominent swelling in the ventral brainstem between the cerebral peduncles of the midbrain cranial to it and the medulla oblongata caudal to it. A furrow for the basilar artery divides the pons into two large convex ridges. The skeletal floor of the pons is the sphenoid bone. The single fourth ventricle lies in the space between the pons and the cerebellum.

Observe the paired cranial nerves leaving the pontine region. The trigeminal (V), which is the largest cranial nerve, is at its cephalic border. The abducent (VI), facial (VII) and vestibulocochlear (VIII) nerves leave the caudal borders of the pons, in successive order.

Locate the cerebellum ((Figures 6-3 and 6-4). It occupies the space between the occipital lobes of the cerebrum and the dorsal aspect of the medulla oblongata. It is attached to the midbrain rostrally by a pair of superior peduncles, to the pons ventrally by the middle peducles, and to the medulla caudally by the inferior peduncles.

Note that the surface of the cerebellum is greatly increased by ridges called folia which are separated by fissures. The cerebellum has a narrow median part called the vermis and a pair of hemispheres, each directed caudally and laterally. The most caudal aspect of the cerebellum has a flocculonodular lobe which is tucked under the hemispheres. An incision into the cerebellum will reveal an outer gray cortex and an inner white matter.

The cerebellum is importantly involved in speech, especially in the reflex control of the muscle spindles and therefore in automatic postural movements and proprioception.

Locate the medulla oblongata, or most caudal aspect of the hindbrain. This is an enlarged area that leads directly into the spinal cord. Refer to Figure 6-4 (norma basalis) and 6-3 (midsagittal view).

Note on the ventral surface of the medulla the medial ventral fissure which runs the entire length of the medulla. This fissure is continuous caudally with the median anterior (ventral) fissure of the spinal cord and it terminates cranially at the pons. Find on the dorsal surface of the medulla a similar dividing groove called the posterior median fissure. (To avoid confusion, a median longitudinal fissure shown in Figure 6-4 is a groove in the ventral and cranial aspects of the brain dividing the cerebral hemispheres.)

Note on the ventral surface paired prominent eminences, the medullary pyramids. They comprise the bulk of the medulla and they carry motor tracts from brain to spinal cord.

Locate the olive as an ovoid prominences on each lateral aspect of the medulla.

Observe that four pairs of cranial nerves exit from the medulla, the glossopharyngeal, vagus, spinal accessory and hypoglossal. The first three pairs arise in a line just dorsal to the olive. The last pair is ventral to the olive. All originate from rootlets which coalesce to trunks.

III. Localized Areas in the Cerebrum

Localization of function in the cerebrum is a concept that is both vigorously supported and opposed. Localization theory postulates cerebral areas both superficial and deep and even subcerebral. The present Exercise provides, on the supposition that there is cerebral localization, a cursory examination of selected areas on the surface of the cerebrum that may control given kinds of function relevant to speech. In the classical terminology of Brodmann, specific areas were numeralized. Later, these areas were given names descriptive of their postulated function.

Locate the principal motor area (#4) in the precentral convolution just rostral to the fissure of Rolando. This is said to control delicate, isolated, voluntary muscle movements, including those of speech. The control is exerted contralaterally (on the other side of the body).

The premotor area (6) is rostral to the principal motor area. It controls voluntary muscles in terms of mass movements, e.g. swinging of the upper extremity in walking. This is a center for postural adjustments. The area is also said to control the acquisition of specialized motor skills.

The suppressor area is a narrow strip between areas 4 and 6. It may transmit signals through the basal ganglia to inhibit muscle tone.

Just rostral to the premotor area there is a frontal eye field (area 8). It is the origin of the corticomesencephalic tract on each side that carries impulses to the nuclei of cranial nerves III, IV and VI which control muscles moving the eyeball.

The anterior tip of each cerebral hemisphere includes the prefrontal areas (#9, 10, 11 and 12). Localization theory involves these areas in shaping the personality, or individual manner of reacting behaviorally.

Locate the postcentral gyrus just behind the fissure of Rolando. Its anterior section, the somatic sensory area I, allows us to localize touch, pressure, vibrations, and kinesthetic sensations. We can judge such things as mass, shape, and texture. This ability is called stereognosis. The posterior section, somatic sensory area II, involves consciousness of pain and temperature.

In the occiptital lobe, there are visual areas (#17, 18 and 19) around the calcarine fissure. These areas involve recognition of visual shapes and sizes. Lesions in the contiguous visual association areas (#20 and 21) may occur in dyslexia.

In the temporal lobe, the final neurons of the cochlear nerve end in each superior temporal gyrus (Heschl's convolution), areas 41 and 42, and impulses spread into neighboring auditory association areas (#22 and 41) for the interpretation of sounds.

Broca's area (45) in the left cortex, in the inferior frontal convolution, was classically postulated as an important speech center. Lesions therein were claimed to be followed by "pure" motor aphasia. The original claim represents the concept of localization extended to an extreme and dubious limit.

The student is refered to Minckler (1972) for diagrams and photographs of the cerebrum; also to Penfield and Roberts (1959) for a discussion of the neurophysiology of languange and localization of function.

EXERCISE 7

HUMAN CRANIAL NERVES
&
BRAIN AND SPINAL CORD IN THE FROG

OBJECTIVES

The student is asked to review the location and roots of exit of the cranial nerves in an isolated human brain. Secondly, he is asked to learn to test in an elementary way the integrity of these nerves in living human subjects. Thirdly, he is asked to study a brain and the arrangement of spinal nerves in a relatively primitive vertebrate, the frog. The student may thus develop a comprehensive overview of the structure and activities particularly of the peripheral nervous system.

TIME REQUIRED

One or up to two laboratory periods - three to four hours

MATERIALS

Preserved human brains
Trays
Frogs
Dissecting instruments including
 rongeur forceps and trephine
Tuning forks and pure tone
 audiometers

Diethyl ether, for anesthesia
Sugar, salt, vinegar, quinine and
 ammonia solutions
Laryngeal mirrors, head mirrors
 and tongue depressors

DESCRIPTION AND PROCEDURE

Re-examine preserved human brain specimens to find the roots of the cranial nerves. Use a standard textbook of anatomy plus the illustrations and keys in Exercise 6 on the brain. Refer also to Figure 7-1.

Tabular Survey of Human Cranial Nerve Function

In the following chart the student is to write the following information: (a) the names of cranial nerves indicated by the numbers provided; and (b) the location of the cranial exit of each nerve.

	Name	Place of Exit
I.		
II.		
III.		
IV.		
V.		
VI.		
VII.		
VIII.		
IX.		
X.		
XI.		
XII.		

Duplicate this chart, listing the cranial nerves in vertical sequence as above. In a second column marked Distribution, write in the correct distribution of each nerve.

FIGURE 7-1
CLOSEUP OF BASE OF THE HUMAN BRAIN SHOWING CRANIAL NERVES

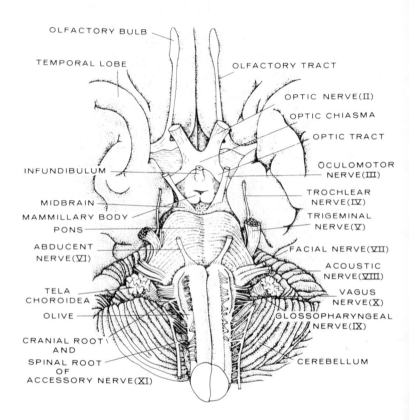

Place each of the following terms opposite the name of the cranial nerve whose distribution it represents:

Abdominal and thoracic viscera
"Chewing" muscles
Extrinsic eye muscles
Internal ear
Iris
Muscles of facial expression
Nasal mucosa
Retina

Skin of face and scalp
Sternocleidomastoid and trapezius muscles
Teeth
Tongue and pharynx (muscles)
Tongue muscles
"Swallowing" muscles (of pharynx)

Make a third chart, again listing the cranial nerves in vertical sequence. In a second column marked Function, place each of the following terms opposite the name of each cranial nerve whose function it represents:

Chewing movements	Sensations of teeth
Equilibrium	Sense of smell
Eye movements	Shoulder movements
Facial expressions	Slowing of heart
Hearing	Swallowing
Movements of tongue	Taste
Peristalsis	Vision
Sensations of scalp and face	

Testing Selected Human Cranial Nerves by Non-Invasive Procedures

Sensory responses whose integrity is of interest to speech pathologists have been selected for study. The students are to descriptively record responses of members of the group and to roughly compare these responses with those of other groups.

It is not feasible to draw firm conclusions about the relative inadequacies of any system tested since the student is not sufficiently sophisticated to set up quantitative response scales to grade the efficiency of the response. The goal here is to present some diverse procedures so that the student may appreciate certain diagnostic evaluations which are practicable and which are readily performed by clinicians.

An unexpected deviation in response, whether motor or sensory, should not lead to the inference that it must be a given nerve that is at fault. There are many elements in a stimulus-response system, any one element of which may malfunction. Do the testing herein with this in mind and also keep in mind that batteries of tests are used clinically.

Cranial Nerve V - Trigeminal

The trigeminal nerve provides for sensation originating from stimuli over the face and part of the scalp. It also controls movement of the mandible. The nerve is mixed (motor and sensory). It has three great divisions, ophthalmic, maxillary and mandibular.

The ophthalmic division can be tested by trying to elicit the corneal reflex, using a hair as the stimulus. The subject should blink bilaterally. If there is no response, ask whether the stimulus was felt. Outline the reflex pathway.

Test the sensory system from the facial skin. This may involve all three divisions of the trigeminal nerve, depending upon the area of the face stimulated. Use cotton wool for touch sensations and pin-pricking for pain sensations. Ask the subject with his eyes closed to distinguish between light pressure and pinprick sensations. Outline the receptors, afferent fibers, and the region of the central nervous system affected.

Test motor aspects of the mandibular division of the trigeminal nerve. Have the subject clench his teeth while you palpate the masseter and temporal muscles to determine the muscle bulk and the force of the contractions. These muscles are supplied by the masseteric and temporal branches.

Two of the several depressor muscles of the mandible, i.e. the mylohoid and anterior belly of the digastric, are supplied by the mylohoid branch of the mandibular nerve. Ask the subject to open his mouth widely. Weakness in the nerve-muscle systems involved is manifested by deviation of the jaw to the weak side or by incapacity for full depression.

The mandibular nerve supplies the medial and lateral pterygoid muscles. The lateral pterygoid is the chief protractor of the jaw, but the medial pterygoid is also involved. The medial pterygoid assists the masseter to elevate the mandible. Ask the subject to perform the motions above, against the opposing force of your fingers.

In any of the tests above, there are sex differences in the force of response. To obtain a sense of what is normal, the examiner must familiarize himself with the nature of the expected responses in a number of healthy subjects. This comes best only with long practice.

Cranial Nerve VII - Facial

The facial nerve has an intimate geographic relation to the middle ear and it gives off many of its branches in the temporal area. Many of its branches innervate the muscles of facial expression. A branch called the nervus intermedius carries sensory fibers for taste from the anterior two-thirds of the tongue and secretomotor fibers to the lacrimal and salivary glands. The facial nerve carries afferent fibers which are thought to be proprioceptive from the expressive muscles and/or which transmit deep pain from the tissues of the face. There is actually very little proprioception or kinesthesia from the facial region. The facial nerve can readily be functionally tested and most tests involve responsiveness of the facial muscles.

Observe any facial asymmetries. Does one side of the mouth droop? Ask your laboratory partner to show his teeth, then puff out his cheeks, whistle, wrinkle his forehead while gazing upward, frown, and close his eyes tightly. Try to open the subject's closed eyes manually. Is one palpebral fissure wider than the other? Test the orbicularis oris muscle by trying to open the subject's lips while he presses them tightly together. Test the platysma muscle by asking the subject to forcibly depress the corners of his mouth; this muscle then usually contracts.

Test the integrity of the lacrimal system by presenting ammonia fumes to the subject's nostrils. Do tear secretions occur?

Test the sense of taste by having the subject protrude his tongue and placing sugar, salt, vinegar and quinine in that order on its anterior two-thirds. Have the subject report what kind of substance he believes he is tasting.

In lesions of the greater petrosal branch, testing shows considerable decrease in lacrimation. If the stapedius muscle is affected, there is painful sensitivity to ordinary sounds. If the chorda tympani branch is involved, taste on the anterior tongue may be lost. If the nerve to the digastric muscle is involved, the mandible and tongue deviate to one side on maximal depression.

Compare individual results that you have recorded with the results of all members of the class.

Cranial Nerve VIII - Cochlear Division

The chief manifestation of disease in the cochlear division of the vestibulocochlear nerve is deafness. Historically, the hearing was tested, and crudely so, by the subject's ability to hear the whispered voice or a ticking watch at given distances. If by any valid test a hearing loss is found, it has to be differentially diagnosed whether it is due to conduction difficulties in the middle ear or to sensori-neural malfunction. In sensori-neural loss, the damage may be in the cochlea of the internal ear, or in the auditory nerve, or both. The nerve tends to be damaged only in certain instances, e.g. in acoustic neuroma (a tumor), or by poisoning with a toxic chemical or drug.

Refer to Exercise 23 which deals with (1) classical tuning fork procedures for helping to identify conduction deafness, and (2) the pure tone audiometer which quantitatively evaluates auditory sensitivity and the degree of hearing loss. There are other kinds of audiometers which need not be considered in this text. The student may delay such testing at this point and initiate an auditory evaluation when Exercise 23 is undertaken.

Cranial Nerve IX - Glossopharyngeal

The ninth cranial nerve is afferent from the tongue and pharynx and efferent to the parotid salivary gland and stylopharyngeus muscle.

Test the receptors and lingual afferents by evaluating the sensation of taste on the posterior third of the tongue which is the region innervated by the lingual branch of the ninth nerve. Apply quinine as the stimulus. The tongue root is especially sensitive to bitter substances in solution and the receptors should be readily stimulated.

Test the pharyngeal receptors and sensory afferents by touching the posterior wall of the subject's pharynx with a tongue depressor. The response should be contraction of the pharyngeal muscles, usually with gagging. The finding in the literature of a persistent gag reflex after experimental section of the ninth nerve in animals suggests that the pharyngeal wall is also supplied by the tenth cranial nerve which makes this test unreliable to evaluate the ninth nerve alone.

Test the integrity of the swallowing reflexes by having the subject drink water. Swallowing involves the pharynx and esophagus, territories supplied by both glossopharyngeal and vagus nerves.

Cranial Nerve X - Vagus

The vagus is a mixed nerve which is distributed extensively to the head, neck, thorax and abdomen. It supplies afferent and efferent fibers to the pharynx and larynx, thus having great importance in speech. The quality of the voice is one index of the integrity of the nerve, although quality is not simply a laryngeal phenomenon.

The condition of the nerve-muscle system to the larynx, particularly with regard to the recurrent laryngeal branch of the vagus, is ascertainable by several kinds of instrumental analysis. In Exercise 16, the student is asked to visualize the normal structure and movements of the true vocal folds, under supervision, by indirect laryngoscopy. Refer to that Exercise if this test is to be performed at this point.

The student need not perform other tests of vagal function, although there are many such tests, e.g. salivary-taste reflex, carotid body relex, cough reflex, gag reflex and vomiting reflex.

Cranial Nerve XI - (Spinal) Accessory

The accessory nerve is formed by the union of a cranial and spinal portion. The student at the start of this Exercise should have seen on the human brain specimen the cranial roots leaving each side of the medulla caudal to the roots of the vagus nerve. The spinal roots arise from the spinal cord, variably from the upper five cervical segments.

The spinal roots unite to produce a nerve that ascends and enters the skull. Both cranial and spinal trunks then descend and unite for a short distance.

The cranial (bulbar) part is often considered to be part of the vagus. By entering the pharyngeal plexus, the cranial sector innervates the soft palate, larynx and constrictors of the pharynx.

The spinal part innervates the sternomastoid and trapezius muscles. Test the spinal part as follows: Ask your laboratory partner to rotate his head forcibly against your hand while you observe and palpate the sternocleidomastoid muscle. Then ask the subject to forcibly elevate (shrug) his shoulders while you palpate the action of both upper trapezii. Next, attempt to depress the subject's shoulders. Test the lower part of the trapezius by having the subject brace his shoulder backward and downward. Weakness in the trapezius is evidenced by a relative difficulty in elevating and retracting the shoulders or in elevating the arms above the horizontal level.

Evaluate the upper, bulbar portion of the eleventh nerve. Select for testing the levator palati nerve-muscle system and observe the movement of the soft palate in a subject who is phonating /i/ as in bEEt. Unilateral weakness (of nerve or muscle) is indicated by failure of the palate to elevate on the disordered side whereas elevation does occur on the healthy side.

In another test of the bulbar section (perhaps complicated by pharyngeal branches of the vagus), ask the subject to say /a/ (ah). The uvula should travel backward in the medial plane.

Cranial Nerve XII - Hypoglossal

Ask the subject to protrude his tongue and to move it rapidly in and out of the mouth or to wiggle it from side to side.An upper motor neuron lesion (pyramidal or extrapyramidal) may cause some contralateral loss of function, although the hypoglossal nerve on each side is claimed to receive upper motor neuron impulses from both sides of the cerebral cortex. A bilateral upper motor neuron lesion will cause the alternate motion of the tongue to be slow. When the lower motor neuron, or hypoglossal nerve proper, is involved, the protruded tongue tends to deviate toward the side of the lesion and atrophy may be manifested by wrinkling of the tongue and loss of tissues on the affected side. Ask the subject to curl his tongue upward in an attempt to touch his nose, and then downward to lick his lower lip. Instruct him to push out his cheek on each side while you as examiner test the strength of his tongue by pushing against it through the bulging cheek.

In another evaluation of the hypoglossal nerve, ask the subject to say "Kitty Tucker," slowly at first, and then to accelerate to the highest rate possible. Persons with a coordination problem in the tongue will reveal it in a failure of diadochokinesis. It should be noted that the failure may be central, presumptively cerebellar primarily, rather than in the hypoglossal nerve.

Dissection of the Frog Brain

Despite some doubt that arises, comparative anatomy has much to offer. The relative uniformity of structures in all vertebrate animals and the orderly and developing complexity from fish to mammal and man bring a unique dimension in reasoning about structure, function and certain kinds of pathology.

In the following dissection, the brain and spinal cord can be seen in much simpler forms than in man and they are thus more easily understood structurally.

Put a live frog in a jar containing ether-soaked absorbent cotton. This is an appropriate method of euthanasia.

Expose the entire dorsal aspect of the brain by chipping away the overlying skull and bones with rongeur forceps and trephine. (The instructor needs to demonstrate these instruments.)

Identify each of the structures shown in Figure7-2. Between the eyes is the cerebrum. Behind the eyes are the optic lobes which connect the optic nerves with the eyes. Between the optic lobes, the pituitary gland rests, surrounded by a stalk, the infundibulum. At the caudal end of the head region, the medulla oblongata lies.

FIGURE 7-2
DISSECTION OF THE FROG'S CENTRAL NERVOUS SYSTEM

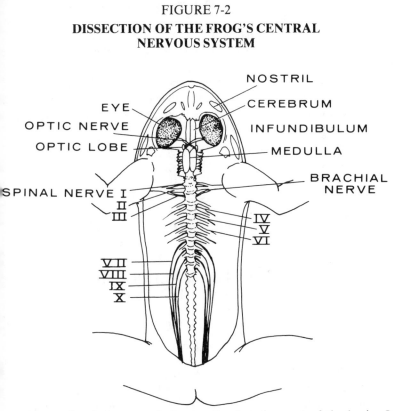

Locate the thalamencephalon on the dorsal aspect of the brain. It lies between the cerebral hemispheres and the optic lobes. The thalamencephalon roughly corresponds to the thalamus in man. Find the cerebellum, a small body between the optic lobes and the medulla.

Note the linear arrangement of the forebrain, midbrain and hindbrain and the absence of flexures. Also note the small size of the cerebrum.

Spinal Nerves in the Frog

To find the spinal nerves, open the chest and abdominal cavity with surgical scissors and remove all visceral organs which obscure the dorsally situated spinal cord.

There are only 10 pairs of spinal nerves in the frog. Locate them with the aid of Figure 7-2.

The second pair of spinal nerves is large and it is joined by fibers from nerves 1 and 3. Their roots combine to form the brachial nerve to the upper extremities.

The fourth, fifth and sixth spinal nerves are small. They innervate chiefly the lateral abdominal aspects of the body.

The remaining four pairs of nerves unite to form the sciatic nerve to the legs. Nerves 8, 9 and 10 are large.

EXERCISE 8

TESTS OF SENSORY PERCEPTION
GENERAL SENSES

OBJECTIVES

In certain speech disorders there may be losses in the sensory sphere. One kind of function that can readily be tested by a beginner non-invasively involves the modalities of (1) skin perception (touch, pain and temperature), and (2) deep perception (sense of position, motion, spatial discrimination and localization, and vibration).

TIME REQUIRED

One laboratory period - two hours

MATERIALS

Mechanical compasses
with movable legs(prongs)
Balance
Small gram weights, pellets and
containers

Pencils with fine points
Electronic stimulators or induction
coils
Tuning forks
Beakers

DESCRIPTION AND PROCEDURE

Cutaneous Receptors

Tactile Discrimination

The subject sits down, closes his eyes, and puts his hand on the table. Apply gently and simultaneously to the back of his hand the two points of a small compass whose prongs are separated by about 5 mm. The subject states whether he feels one or two points. Change the point distances gradually, applying them to the same area until a change in sensation is obvious. The minimum distance where the two points are individually sensed is the threshold expressed as tactile discrimination in mm. Obtain values for the palm, finger tips, lips, and both surfaces of the forearm. Compare thresholds among members of your group.

Tactile Localization

Press the tip of a pencil firmly down upon some skin region so as to leave an impression. The subject with eyes closed tries to duplicate this position with a pencil. The distance between the two impressions is measured. Do this for the lips, finger tips, palm of hand and both surfaces of the forearm.

Distribution: Mark the pressure spots on the surface of the skin, using a restricted area. Stimulate lightly with a hair.

Weber's Law

The subject closes his eyes and places his hand, palm up, on the table. Place on the distal phalanges of his index and middle fingers a box containing shot (10 grams). Once the subject states that he feels the weight, add shot until the smallest increment is just perceived. Record the increment.

Repeat, starting with 20, 30, 40 and 50 grams, respectively. In each case note the increment of shot added before the subject perceives the difference. If the subject just feels a one gram increment starting at 10 gm, he may just sense a 2 gram increment starting at 20 gm, a 3 gram increment at 30 gm, and so on up.

The "law" states that equal relative differences are equally perceptible. If true, the ratios in each trial should be all about the same. The law holds roughly and only for medium ranges. It also holds roughly for other sensations. It suggests that we distinguish intensity differences by relative and not by absolute differences.

The student should be asked to do reading in standard textbooks of physiology and psychology concerning controversies about the above principle, particularly with regard to the visual sensation.

Pain

Punctiform Distribution: Limit an area about 3 cm square on the back of the forearm. Soak it in warm water to soften the skin. Examine the area point by point, by pressing a needle firmly upon the skin without piercing it. Mark the pain spots for surface identification. Are pain spots coincident with pressure spots? Referring to standard textbooks in physiology, outline the separate pathways for crude touch, discriminative touch and pain, from receptors to terminal endings on the cerebrum.

Threshold Value: Arrange an electronic stimulator or classical induction coil for single shocks. Lightly touch the electrodes to the tip of the tongue. Start with very weak voltage. Increase the stimulus intensity just to where the threshold for pain is reported. Determine the threshold for other regions, e.g. the skin of the forearm. Stimulate with shocks increasing above the threshold and note that the value for just perceiving pain is not the same as that for which pain is distinct.

Temperature

Test the temperature sense by touching a subject whose eyes are closed with a metal object. The subject should perceive the object as cool.

Deep Receptors

Proprioception

Although proprioceptive impulses and adjustment are important in the maintenance of posture and the control of movement, even extensive defects can be concealed by compensatory use of other sensory systems, chiefly the eyes.

Romberg's Sign

Unmask any relevant latent defect in proprioception by having the subject perform the following activity with his eyes shut. Have the subject stand up with his heels together. A normal person will often sway, but will rarely fall. Violent swaying and fall are termed a "positive" Romberg. In that instance the afferent systems relaying impulses from the soles of the feet and muscles of the lower extremities are not sending appropriate informational signals concerning particularly the length and tension of the muscles and their positions in space. There may also be a disorder of the labyrinth of the ear or the vestibular nerve system.

Have the subject stand on one leg with his eyes closed. A normal young person can accomplish it, although usually with noticeable sway. This is an unreasonable test in the elderly.

Test the position sense in another way by placing your hand in a given posture. Ask the subject to imitate that position. Also have him position your other hand identically. An inability to do these tasks suggests a disturbance of the position sense.

Continue testing by moving a blindfolded subject's finger up and down several times, stopping in the elevated or depressed position. Have the subject state whether the finger is up or down. There should normally be no loss of the proprioceptive clues.

Cerebellar Involvement in Postural Activity

The act of walking requires information from cutaneous and deep receptors and it also involves normal brain function.

Test the subject's ability to walk along a straight line on the floor. Any dyscoordination (ataxia) is not influenced by closing the eyes if the cerebellum is involved. Closing the eyes would influence the presence of cerebral ataxia.

Static Ataxia

Have the subject touch alternately, slowly and rapidly, the tip of his nose with the tip of one of his fingers. An ataxic tremor should not be evident if the subject is normal.

Dysmetria (Inability to Measure Distance)

Elicit any relevant abnormality by asking the subject to raise his arms and bring them quickly to a stop at the horizontal level. If dysmetric, one arm may drop below the level.

Check for ataxia and dysmetria by asking the subject to lift a glass of water to his lips. If there is cerebellar ataxia, the movement of the upper extremity may not be steady or well timed.

Dyssynergia

Have the subject perform rapidly successive antagonistic movements, such as pronation and supination of the palm of the hand. Observe the responses. Repeated and marked failure to perform reciprocal movements is termed adiadochokinesis. Test this also by asking the subject to say "buttercup" rapidly. This involves rapid protusive and retractive positional changes of the tongue.

Coordination and Past-Pointing

The subject, with eyes open, sits opposite the observer, stretches out his right arm directly in front and touches the observer's finger with his own index finger. He then closes his eyes and moves his arm back until it is pointing to the right. He next attempts to return the arm to its former position, with his index finger touching the observer's finger. The subject is to repeat this test in a vertical plane, because a failure may occur in one plane and not in another. If the subject cannot touch the observer's finger, but his finger comes to rest some distance away, this is called past-pointing.

Stereognosis

Stereognosis is the recognition of the three-dimensional aspects (shape, form, etc.) of objects by touch. With objects having much weight, or pressed into the palm of the hand, deep as well as cutaneous receptors are usually stimulated. (Perception of weight is called barognosis.)

Have the subject, with eyes closed, name and describe objects such as a penknife, a rubber band, a piece of string, and also objects of other geometric shapes, textures and weights. The size, shape, use and name should be stated. The object must not be touched with the other hand. Failures are classified as astereognosis. This signifies a postcentral sensory cortical, or subcortical loss.

Vibration Sensibility (Pallesthesia)

Test the vibration sense by applying the base of a vibrating tuning fork of low pitch (not greater than 128 Hz) to a subcutaneous bony prominence. Record the time that the subject says the sensation persists. Compare both sides of the body; inequality of duration suggests some loss of the vibratory sense. Test in succession, bones of the fingers, radial styloid and external malleolus.

With the subject's eyes closed, repeat the test using only the fingers.

EXERCISE 9

ACTION POTENTIALS IN FROG SCIATIC NERVES

OBJECTIVES

The bodily organs intercommunicate by signals. Chemical signals involve chiefly hormones which diffuse throughout the body to definite targets. The action is slow, but sustained. Neural signals involve electrochemical transmission, or action potentials. These are very fast, but die away quickly. In the present experiment, the nature of action potentials is stressed.

TIME REQUIRED

One laboratory period - two hours

MATERIALS

Electronic stimulators
Cathode ray oscilloscopes or
   strip chart recorders
Preamplifiers
Cables

Nerve chambers
Dissecting instruments, trays,
   beakers, glass rods, and
   surgical ligatures
Ringer's solution (cold-blooded)
Frogs

DESCRIPTION

Conduction of signals in a single neuron occurs in all directions. The signals, which are electrochemical currents, are conducted in jumps (saltatory conduction) along the neuron. This is because the fatty myelin sheath covering the neuron is interrupted periodically by nodes of Ranvier. The impulse transmission occurs from node to node.

At rest, a potential difference exists between the inside and outside of the fiber. The fiber is polarized, the potential difference inside being about minus 85 mv with respect to the outside.

Upon stimulation, the membrane depolarizes at the nodes and sodium ions rapidly move inside. Potassium ions move out. The potential inside reverses and may reach about + 35 mv relative to the outside. Upon membrane repolarization, the ions reverse their directional flows and an absolute refractory period of rest occurs.

The state of excitation travels across synapses to the next neuron. Excitation is unidirectional because the energy sources are on the presynaptic neuron and the receptors are on the postsynaptic neuron.

The axon fires according to the all-or-none law once it has responded to a minimal stimulus intensity. It fires maximally or not at all.

The student should read standard physiology texts to visualize the form of various kinds of potentials in man.

Summation

There are many nerve fibers in a gross nerve. Each, many, or all can be stimulated.

Spatial Summation

This occurs when a number of fibers fire together. Stimulating more and more of these fibers increases the strength of the response until the maximum response occurs because all the fibers are activated.

Temporal Summation

This occurs when the frequency of impulses increases in a neuron and its fibers.

PROCEDURE

Set up a system (Figure 9-1) to stimulate the moist sciatic nerve of a frog that has been pithed and then carefully dissected. Use glass rods on the nerve rather than metal probes. Get the longest possible length of nerve before freeing it from the body. Place the nerve in a beaker with cold-blooded Ringer's solution.

FIGURE 9-1
STIMULATING SYSTEM TO ELICIT
ACTION POTENTIALS IN FROG NERVE

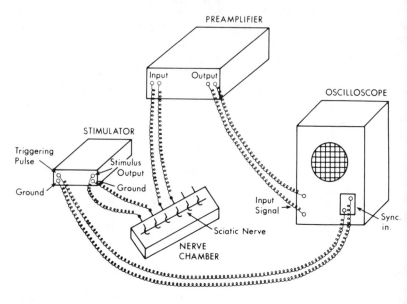

Connect the stimulator and oscilloscope by a ground lead and a triggering pulse lead which synchronize the stimulus and the sweep on the oscilloscope. In switching manually there are difficulties in applying multiple stimuli.

Place a moist thread (substituting for the nerve) over a moist towel in a nerve chamber. Insert the moist thread in the chamber over a series of hooks.

Adjust the oscilloscope vertical gain control to 5 mV/cm and the sweep time to 2 msec/cm.

Set the stimulator to 0.1 volt (duration of 1 msec) and stimulus frequency to 60/sec.

Obtain a signal from the thread, adjusting the stimulus voltage to get good visibility. The signal is a stimulus artifact as a result of transmission down the thread. This is not the same as the action potential which will be excited in the neuron.

Substitute the nerve, laying it over the hooks. Connect the nerve to the oscilloscope by two leads which are shielded, with no ground attached. Connect the stimulator to the nerve by two leads, one of which is a ground lead. It may be necessary to place a preamplifier between the nerve and the oscilloscope.

Adjust the oscilloscope roughly as stated above. Starting at 0.1 mV, increase the voltage until an action potential is seen. What is the threshold voltage? Repeat this process several times to obtain an average value.

Apply a single adequate stimulus pulse and note the appearance of the action potential. Increase the stimulus frequency in steps and watch on the oscilloscope screen any alterations in the action potential.

With the stimulator and oscilloscope at optimal values, observe the action potential on the screen. Determine the voltage, frequency and time from the stimulus artifact at which the action potential begins.

EXERCISE 10

ELECTROENCEPHALOGRAM IN MAN

OBJECTIVES

The student should appreciate the applicability of the electroencephalogram (EEG) to the analysis of neural behavior. Electroencephalography has been stated to be a useful procedure in the study of language-related neurophysiologic processes (Lass, 1976). Regardless of whether this claim stands the test of time, an overview of the use of possible relevant instruments, including a sense of their advantages and limitations, can well be included in the training of the student. This Exercise requires considerable supervision, but under such circumstances it is informative. Interpretation of the record (EEG) requires far more sophistication than the beginner is expected to have and it is here that instructional expertise is essential.

TIME REQUIRED

One laboratory period - two hours

Materials

Miniature skin electrodes   Bio-amplifier
Ear clip electrodes   Channel recorder
Conductive electrode cream   Shielded cables

DESCRIPTION

The electroencephalogram expresses in visual recording the electrical activity within the brain. The records are obtained from specialized electrodes placed on the surface of the scalp. The waveforms that are seen represent a summation of potentials coming from an extremely large number of neurons in the vicinity of the electrodes. The electrical patterns may be a result of graded potentials in the dendrites of neurons in the cerebral cortex and in other parts of the brain. All-or-none action potentials are hardly if at all involved.

PROCEDURE

There are several types of scalp electrodes, including pads, discs, "stick-on" electrodes and needle electrodes, all applied differently. Surface electrodes which are small discs about 7 mm in diameter are satisfactory for the present study. These miniature skin electrodes are not the same as the large, flat, plate electrodes used in electrocardiography. Attach only two of the electrodes (+ and −) high on the forehead, one on the right and the other on the left. Before applying the electrodes, rub the underlying skin vigorously and apply conductive electrode cream to the skin sites selected. Seat the electrodes firmly to avoid artifacts.

The number of electrodes placed on the head for routine clinical recording is variable but may be about 20. The present study is greatly simplified. Also, there are internationally recognized positions for the placement of scalp electrodes.

A ground reference electrode is necessary to reduce electrical noise. This is a special clip electrode which can be placed on one ear lobe of the subject.

To improve the quality of the biologic signals, connect the electrodes to a bio-amplifier. (One example is Model 631 Bio-Amplifier, AC coupled, Phipps and Bird, from Fisher Scientific Company, 711 Forbes Avenue, Pittsburgh, PA 15219. Any good commercial model can be selected which augments signals in the millivolt or microvolt range.) Set the bio-amplifier at an appropriate sensitivity, e.g. 50 microvolts/cm.

Connect the output of the amplifier to a channel recorder (Physiograph or other models). The cable to the recorder should be shielded.

Have the subject in dorsal recumbency. Obtain a record for at least 30 seconds, at low paper speed (15mm/sec), with the subject's eyes closed. Repeat this at a paper speed of 30 mm/sec. A time scale can be placed on the record by a time-marker pen generated by a pulse of one mark per second.

Have the subject keep his eyes open and obtain a record at a paper speed of 30 mm/sec. Repeat this alternation a few times. Are there any noticeable differences in the records?

With the subject's eyes open, record a series of waves, each series for about 30 seconds. Then have the subject do simple arithmetic problems without his resorting to writing. Obtain records during this mental activity and for a few seconds thereafter. Note any changes in the tracing.

Take a sequence of records with the subject breathing deeply and regularly at a rate of about 20 breaths per minute for two minutes. Place emphasis upon forced expiration. Avoid excess paleness of the subject, which could lead to fainting. The usual indication in the EEG of pathologic effects of hyperventilation is the appearance of slowed electrical waves.

Observe the major features of the various EEG records as follows:

1. The most persistent rhythm - alpha ordinarily
2. The presence of delta, beta or theta rhythms
3. Episodes of spikes and whether of long or short duration
4. Background activity

REFERENCES

Exercise 5

Crouch, J. E. **Functional Human Anatomy.** 28th edition, Philadelphia: Lea and Febiger, 1973.

Francis, C. C. **Introduction to Human Anatomy.** 6th edition. St. Louis: The C. V. Mosby Company, 1973.

Grollman, S. **A Laboratory Manual of Mammalian Anatomy and Physiology.** New York: The Macmillan Company, 1964.

Exercise 6

Anderson, J. E. **Grant's Atlas of Anatomy.** 7th edition. Baltimore: Williams and Wilkins Company, 1978.

Ford, D.H. Illari, J. and Schade, J. P. **Atlas of the Human Brain.** 3rd edition. New York: Elsevier Publishing Company, 1978.

McMinn, R. M. H. and Hutchings, R. T. **Color Atlas of Human Anatomy.** Chicago: Year Book Medical Publishers, 1977.

Minckler, J. **Introduction to Neuroscience.** St. Louis: C. V. Mosby Company, 1972.

Penfield, W. and Roberts, L. **Speech and Brain: Mechanisms.** Princeton: Princeton University Press, 1959.

Truex, R. C. and Carpenter, M. B. **Human Neuroanatomy.** Baltimore: Williams and Wilkins Company, 1969.

Exercise 7

Gilroy, J. and Meyer, J.S. **Medical Neurology.** 2nd Edition. New York: Macmillan Publishing Company, 1975.

Holmes, S. J. **The Biology of the Frog.** 4th edition. New York: The Macmillan Company, 1934.

Lofts. B (Ed.). **Physiology of the Amphibia.** Volume III. New York: Academic Press, 1976.

Merritt, H. H. **A Textbook of Neurology.** 6th edition. Philadelphia: Lea and Febiger, 1979.

Exercise 8

Guyton, A. C. **Textbook of Medical Physiology.** 5th edition. Philadelphia: W. B. Saunders Company, 1976.

Hopkins, H. U. **Leopold's Principles and Methods of Physical Diagnosis.** 3rd edition. Philadelphia, W. B. Saunders Company, 1965.

Judge, R. D. and Zuidema, G. D. (Eds.). **Physical Diagnosis: A Physiologic Approach to the Clinical Examination.** 2nd edition. Boston: Little, Brown and Company, 1968.

Exercise 9

Cromwell, L., Arditti, M., Labok, J., Pfeiffer, E. A., Steel, B. and Weibell, F. **Medical Instrumentation for Health Care.** New Jersey: Prentice-Hall, Inc., 1976.

Experiments in General Physiology. American Physiological Society, Washington, D.C., 1959.

Guyton, A. C. **Textbook of Medical Physiology.** 5th edition. Philadelphia: W. B. Saunders Company, 1976.

Langley, C. C. **Physiology of Man.** New York: Van Nostrand Reinhold Company,1971.

Ochs, S. **Elements of Neurophysiology.** New York: John Wiley and Sons, Inc. 1965.

Schade, J. P. and Ford, D. H. **Basic Neurology.** New York: Elsevier Publishing Company, 1971.

Exercise 10

Cooper, R., Osselton, J. W. and Shaw, J. C. **EEG Technology.** London: Butterworth and Company, 1969.

Cromwell, L., Arditti, M, Weibell, F. J., Pfeiffer, E. A., Steele, B. and Labok, J. **Medical Instrumentation for Health Care.** Englewood Cliffs, N.J.: Prentice-Hall, Inc., 1976.

Erlanger, J. and Gasser, H. S. **Electrical Signs of Nervous Activity.** 2nd edition. Philadelphia: University of Pennsylvania Press, 1968.

Kooi, K. A. **Fundamentals of Electroencephalography.** San Francisco: Harper and Row, 1971.

Lass, N. J. **Contemporary Issues in Experimental Phonetics.** New York: Academic Press, 1976.

Rudin, S. G., Foldvari, T. L., and Levy, C. K. **Bioinstrumentaion.** Millis, Mass.: Harvard Apparatus Foundation, 1971.

CHAPTER III
Respiratory System

EXERCISE 11

BONES OF THE HUMAN THORACIC CAGE

OBJECTIVES

A knowledge of the bony framework of the thorax, its joints and its muscles can lead to an understanding of the mechanics of the breathing process. The student should extend this knowledge to the role of thoracic structures in breathing for speech.

TIME REQUIRED

One laboratory period - two hours

MATERIALS

Intact skeletons and disarticulated thoracic bones

DESCRIPTION AND PROCEDURE

Refer to the reference texts while examining the intact skeleton. Note the nature of the thoracic bones and how they are joined together. From the texts, sketch roughly the positions of the major superficial and deep muscles which move the thoracic structures in inspiration and in expiration. Visualize on the thoracic cage the 11 pairs of external intercostal and 11 pairs of internal intercostal muscles.

Clavicle (Collar Bone)

Note that the clavicle articulates medially with the manubrium of the sternum and laterally with the acromion process of the scapula. Observe the reverse curvature of the clavicle.

Draw an outline of the clavicle and the positions of muscles on it, i.e. sternomastoid, pectoralis major, trapezius, deltoid, subclavius and sternohyoid.

Discuss clavicular breathing in singing and talking.

Sternum (Breast Bone)

The sternum is a shield-like, flattened bone, forming the ventromedial aspect of the thoracic cage. Observe its shape and its articulations (1) at its superior ends with the clavicles, and (2) along its lateral margins directly with the cartilages of the first seven pairs of ribs. The costal cartilages permit motion of the ribs at their sternal ends during breathing.

The sternum is divided from above downward into three sections fixed together by fibrous joints. The highest is the manubrium, which is a broad, thick, quadrangular bone. The manubrium is convex ventrally and concave dorsally. Of interest, because of respiratory and laryngeal involvement, are the muscles originating from the manubrium, including the pectoralis major, sternomastoid, sternohyoid and sternothyroid. Using the text, sketch these muscles in an outline of the bone. Note on the manubrium, the jugular notch in the superior border, and the facets on the lateral borders for the first two ribs.

Respiratory System

FIGURE 11-1
THORACIC CAGE

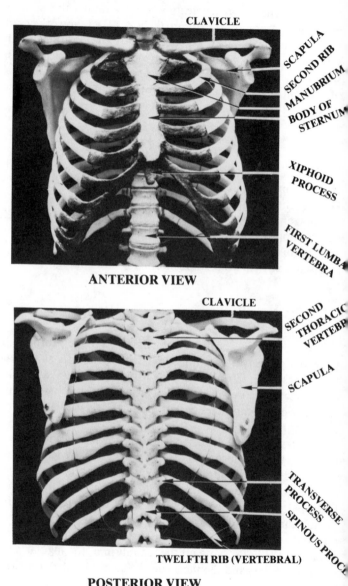

CLAVICLE

SCAPULA

SECOND RIB

MANUBRIUM

BODY OF STERNUM

XIPHOID PROCESS

FIRST LUMBAR VERTEBRA

ANTERIOR VIEW

CLAVICLE

SECOND THORACIC VERTEBRA

SCAPULA

TRANSVERSE PROCESS

SPINOUS PROCESS

TWELFTH RIB (VERTEBRAL)

POSTERIOR VIEW

FIGURE 11-1 (Continued)
THORACIC CAGE

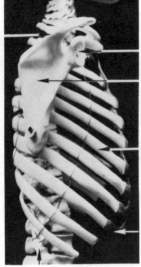

SPINOUS PROCESS OF SCAPULA

GLENOID FOSSA

INFRASPINATOUS PROCESS OF SCAPULA

SIXTH RIB (TRUE RIB)

COSTAL CARTILAGE

TWELFTH RIB (VERTEBRAL)

LATERAL VIEW

The next lower section of the sternum is the corpus, or body. This long, narrow section is widest inferiorly. Its lateral margins show the demifacets for the second costal cartilage and also the facets for costal cartilages of ribs three through seven. In a sketch, show roughly, with the aid of a text, the extent of origin of the pectoralis major muscle.

The lowest sternal part is the xiphoid (ensiform) process. This is a triangular cartilage, its base superior. The xiphoid is frequently seen to be ossified in older specimens. This section is of interest in speech because it affords attachment for the diaphragm, transverse thoracic muscle, and the muscles of the ventral abdominal wall.

FIGURE 11-2
CLAVICLE

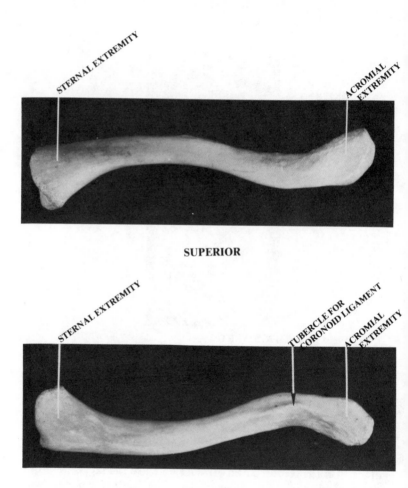

SUPERIOR

INFERIOR

FIGURE 11-3
ANTERIOR VIEW OF
STERNUM AND COSTAL CARTILAGES

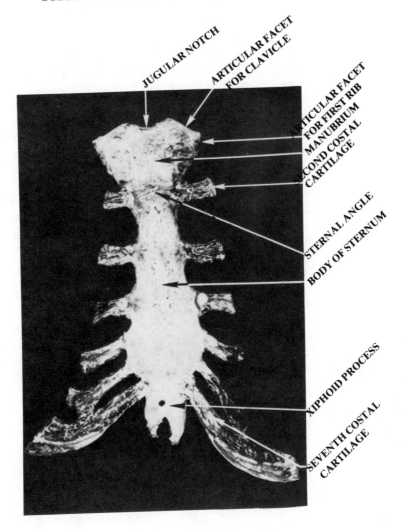

Scapula (Shoulder Blade)

The scapula is a flat, triangular bone, forming the dorsal portion of the shoulder girdle. It articulates with the clavicle and humerus and it provides a broad attachment for several muscles.

Observe the broad concavity (subscapular fossa) of its ventral (costal) surface which overlies the dorsal part of the rib cage. Most of the fossa is filled with the subscapularis muscle.

Examine the dorsal surface. Note its division to two unequal parts by a large spine. The upper section is the supraspinatous fossa and the lower larger section is the infraspinatous fossa.

There are three borders. The concave superior border ends laterally in the scapular notch (or foramen). The very long vertebral border, which extends from the medial to the inferior angle, affords attachment to many muscles. The thick axillary border extends from the glenoid cavity to the inferior angle

The uppermost part of the scapula is the acromion, the broadened lateral extension of its spine. It provides attachment particularly for the deltoid and trapezius muscles.

Observe the shallow, articular surface called the glenoid cavity on the lateral angle of the scapula. The cavity forms a joint with the head of the humerus (arm bone).

Just above the glenoid fossa is a thickened, curved, prominent process, called the coracoid process. It is ventral to the acromion. Its most distal part projects ventrolaterally. Its surfaces are of interest in that they allow insertion of a respiratory muscle, the pectoralis minor. Other muscles, of less relevant interest, are also present.

Ribs (Costae)

The twelve pairs of ribs comprise most of the ventrolateral and dorsolateral part of the thoracic cage. Their elevation in inspiration and depression in expiration are necessary (and especially so in costal breathing) to obtain the pressures and volumes of air used both for breathing and speech. Observe on the whole skeleton how elevation of the ribs could increase the volume of the thoracic cavity during inspiration. The loose attachment of the lower ribs to the sternum permits considerable freedom of movement in the inspiratory phase.

FIGURE 11-4
SCAPULA

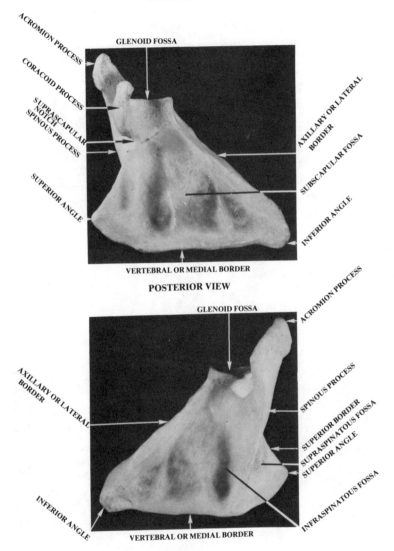

POSTERIOR VIEW

ANTERIOR VIEW

FIGURE 11-5
RIBS

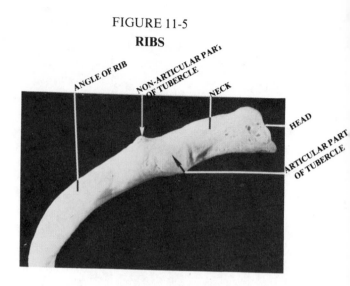

VERTEBRAL END

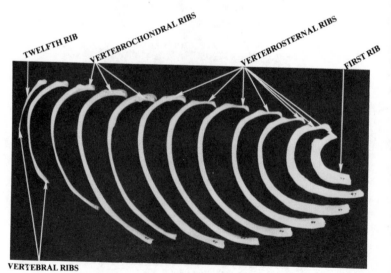

SET OF RIBS

The upper seven ribs are attached via costal cartilages to the sternum. The eighth, ninth and tenth are only indirectly attached to the sternum via the costal cartilages. The last two are incompletely extended ventrally and gain no attachment to the sternum.

Observe on the whole skeleton the nature of the medial attachments of the ribs to the sternum. Note that all twelve ribs are attached dorsally by facets or demifacets to the twelve thoracic vertebrae.

Select a rib from the middle of the series and see that it has a vertebral end, sternal end and a long, curved shaft. At the dorsal (vertebral) extremity, the rib has a head, neck and tubercle. The head articulates with the two demifacets on the bodies of the vertebrae. The tubercle fits into the facet of a transverse process of a vertebra. The neck is the section between the head and tubercle. The shaft is convex externally. At its angle the rib bends in two directions. The concave internal surface has a costal groove just above the lower border which carries the intercostal vessels and nerve. The ventral (sternal) extremity is flattened. It presents a concave depression which receives its costal cartilage.

Thoracic Vertebrae

The thoracic section of the vertebral column is the most relevant section in the respiratory contribution to the speech process because of its position and thus its function in breathing. Cervical vertebrae have the next, but lesser degree of importance.

Each vertebra is distinctive in form, although its structure and classification within a given geographic group are understandable. Study the vertebrae on the intact skeleton. Then examine individual disarticulated vertebrae, emphasizing the thoracic group, but roughly examining the rest of the 26 vertebrae that comprise the human adult vertebral column.

Note that each of the 12 thoracic vertebrae has a slightly heartshaped body. Angled laterally, just dorsal to the body, are the right and left transverse processess. Each process contains a facet to articulate with the tubercles of the ribs. A pair of pillar-like pedicles extends dorsally from the body. A pair of roofing plates, or laminae, run from the pedicles to join in V-shaped fashion more dorsally. From the apex of the V the blended laminae produce a spinous process

FIGURE 11-6
THORACIC VERTEBRA

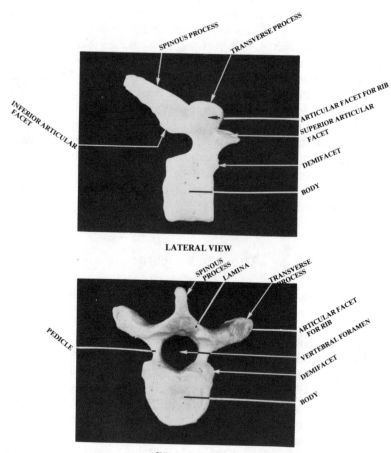

LATERAL VIEW

INFERIOR VIEW

which angles dorsoinferiorly to a somewhat pointed extremity. The thinness and angulation of the spinous process help identify a thoracic vertebra.

Observe that in addition to the facet on the transverse processes for articulation with rib tubercles, the head of the rib also articulates with a facet on the body of the vertebra. This facet is formed by union of an inferior demifacet on the vertebra just above with a superior demifacet of the vertebra just below the one in question. These demifacets also help identify the thoracic vertebrae.

EXERCISE 12

AIR COLUMN REQUIREMENTS AND SPEECH

OBJECTIVES

During phonation there must be an adequate volume and pressure of subglottic air, delivered at controlled rates. The volume expended depends upon factors such as the sound and its position in the word.

The spirometer is a classical instrument to measure lung volumes. It is particularly useful as a basic teaching tool, although it is inefficient for clinical use in speech studies. Spirometry does not solve questions about the relationship of respiratory volumes and speech or how the lung volumes are organized and utilized in speech. The knowledge of various volumes of air passing through the airways is nevertheless important to know despite the lack of immediate applicability and the student is asked to become familiar with spirometers and to determine respiratory volumes and capacities.

TIME REQUIRED

One laboratory period - two hours

MATERIALS

Spirometers: dial and pen recording
Nose clamps

70% ethyl alcohol for sterilization of mouthpieces

DESCRIPTION

The dial-recording, wet spirometer (Figure 12-1) consists of a tank inverted in another tank which is filled with water. The inverted tank is counterbalanced by a weight so that its own weight appears to be zero. By mouthpiece and tubing, the subject can either inhale from or exhale into the tank, thus causing it to fall or rise. The amount of air inhaled or exhaled can be read or calculated from an indicator on the spirometer.

Volume data fall into the following classifications:

A. Pulmonary Volumes

1. Tidal volume : The volume of air moved with each quiet breath
2. Inspiratory reserve volume : The volume of air that can be inspired by forceful inspiration in addition to the tidal volume
3. Expiratory reserve volume : The volume of air that can be forcefully expired after tidal expiration
4. Residual volume : The volume of air remaining in the lungs after the most forceful expiration

B. Pulmonary Capacities

1. Inspiratory capacity : Tidal volume plus inspiratory reserve volume
2. Functional residual capacity : Expiratory reserve volume plus residual volume
3. Vital capacity : Tidal volume plus inspiratory reserve volume plus expiratory reserve volume
4. Total lung capacity: Sum of the four pulmonary volumes.

PROCEDURE

Dial-Recording Spirometer

1. After raising the bell to the 1.5 liter mark, the subject with his nose clamped should breathe normally into the spirometer about fifteen times. Add the volumes of the last ten "normal" breaths, then divide the sum by ten. This gives the subject's average tidal

FIGURE 12-1
SPIROMETER: DIAL RECORDING

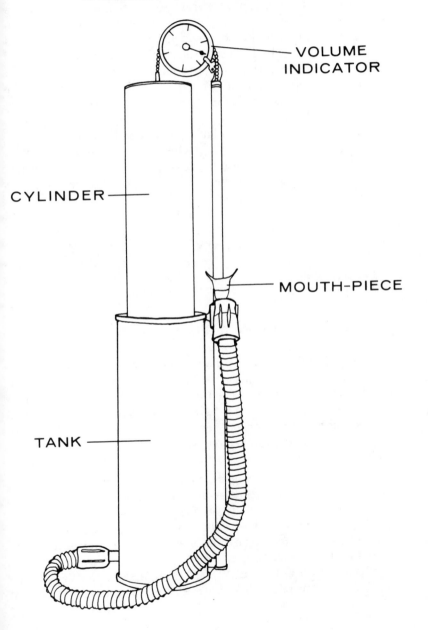

volume (TV).

2. Reset the indicator to zero and let the subject take several normal breaths without the spirometer tube in his mouth. At the end of a normal expiration, the subject should blow as much air as he can into the tube. This procedure should be repeated several times and an average taken. This is the expiratory reserve volume (ER).

3. After the subject rests for a few minutes, have him inhale as deeply as possible and then maximally force all the air he can into the spirometer. Read this expired volume and record it as the vital capacity (VC).

4. The inspiratory reserve volume (IR) can be found by having the subject inspire as deeply as possible through the mouth. He then makes only a normal (not forced) expiration into the spirometer. Subtract the tidal air volume and consider the remainder as the inspiratory reserve volume.

Calculate the following from the data:

Inspiratory capacity   =   TV + IR
Functional residual capacity =   ER + RV*
Total lung capacity   =   RV + ER + IR + RV

(*Residual volume cannot be measured by the spirometric procecure used above. For the present purposes, use   a textbook value for age and sex.)

Pen-Recording Spirometer

A pen-recording spirometer measures the flow of air in a given time and it is a common instrument used for dynamic clinical measurements of pulmonary function. The Collins 13.5 liter spirometer (Warren Collins Co., Braintree, MA 02184) is an acceptable, watersealed spirometer with direct writing pen. This is a system in which exhaled carbon dioxide is absorbed by soda lime. The pen describes a spirogram (Figure 12-2).

The basic measurements made from the spirogram are tidal volume, inspiratory reserve volume, expiratory reserve volume, vital capacity, and the expiratory volume at the first second of the timed (forced) vital capacity curve (FEV_1). The maximal mid-expiratory air flow (MMEF) taken from the midportion of the VC spirogram is also an important measurement.

Measure the TV, IRV, ERV, VC, FEV_1 and the MMEF. (If only the VC and some related basic volumes are to be determined, the sim-

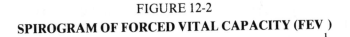

FIGURE 12-2
SPIROGRAM OF FORCED VITAL CAPACITY (FEV$_1$)

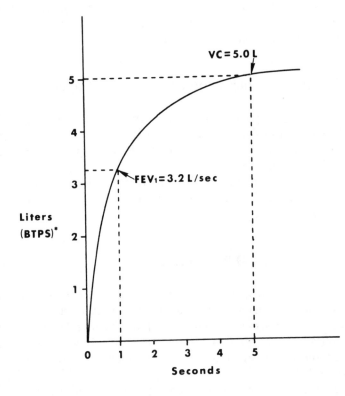

*BTPS refers to volume exhaled and stated by computation to be at body temperature, ambient pressure, and saturated with water vapor at 37°C. The original experimental data were taken at "ambient temperature" and were stated prior to conversion at ATPS.

plified Collins spirometer which records on a dial is satisfactory.) Obtain the TV and VC at slow speed (160 mm/min and the FEV$_1$ at 1920 mm/min (where the distance between two vertical lines is one second).

For the FEV$_1$, examine the record at the one second point for the maximally expired air following maximal inspiration. Time is important and the subject is instructed to exhale not only as hard as he can, but as fast as he can. The FEV$_1$ should be at least 80% of the predicted value for the "forced" vital capacity.

In the 13.5 liter spirometer, multiply all recorded volumes by 2 (which compensates for the large radius of the bell where volume $=\pi r^2 h$ for a cylinder). The data are taken at ATPS (vapor saturated, air temperature and barometric pressure) and they can be converted to BTPS (vapor saturated, body temperature and barometric pressure) by standard tables correcting for any spirometer temperature.

Relation of Voice Production to Vital Capacity

There is no predictable relationship between vital capacity and "good" voice. In ordinary conversational speech only about 20 per cent of the vital capacity is said to be used, although almost all may be used in singing (Wyke, 1974).

Have a subject inhale maximally, then find with a stopwatch how long he can sustain each of a number of different phonemes. Are there differences?

Air-Flow During Speech

There are recent advances in flowmeters to measure air flow rates during speech. The pneumotachograph is a very acceptable device. As air flows across a resistance, there is a fall in pressure related linearly to the volume rate of air flow. The pressure drop is converted by a pressure transducer to an electrical voltage which is in turn amplified and recorded.

The body plethysmograph is becoming of increasing use to study the relationship between pressures, air flow rates, and lung volume during speech as well as breathing (DuBois et al., 1956; Hixon and Warren, 1971).

Demonstrate these instruments, if they are available.

Breath-Holding Test

Have the seated subject exhale once as deeply as possible, then inhale fully and hold his breath as long as possible. The average time of the hold in the young male adult is 65 seconds, the minimum 45 seconds. The average time in the female is 60 seconds. Compare individual with class data.

Expiratory Force Test

Use a glass U-tube manometer, each arm half full of mercury. Have the subject blow the mercury up by exhaling with maximum force. The height to which the mercury is blown averages about 110 mm (in males), with a minimum of 80 mm. Compare individual with class data.

EXERCISE 13

PNEUMOGRAPHY IN MAN

OBJECTIVES

The student is asked to visualize the character of chest movements by pneumography. He should be able by this procedure to record thoracic movements both in normal breathing and speaking.

TIME REQUIRED

One laboratory period - two hours

MATERIALS

Pneumographs, mechanical or
  electronic
Rubber tubing, T-tubes, bulbs,
  and clamps
Marey tambours

Signal magnets
Kymographs
Channel recorders

Electronic pneumographic equipment is commercially available using channel recording systems and it should be utilized in preference to the classical manual recording systems. We have satisfactorily utilized the Physiograph and many of its attachments from Narco Bio-Systems, Inc., 7651 Airport Blvd., Houston, Texas 77017. We find this channel recording system to be satisfactory for student work. There are several other vendors with quality equipment in this field and we do not preferentially endorse any one system.

DESCRIPTION

The pneumograph (mechanical or electronic) registers the movements of the thorax. The mechanical type consists of a coiled spring covered by a rubber tube, and its ends are connected by an adjustible chain. Tubing connects the pneumograph to a Marey tambour, the latter being a metal tube connected to a metal dish with a rubber membrane closing the dish. The system is filled with air and

FIGURE 13-1
ELECTRONIC PNEUMOGRAPH

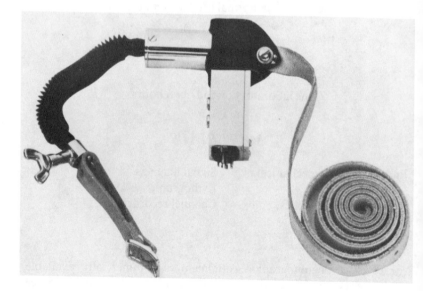

closed to the atmosphere. When the pneumograph is stretched or compressed, the change in volume alters the pressure of air within the system. As a result the rubber membrane over the tambour is elevated or depressed. A writing stylus whose base rests on the membrane is correspondingly elevated or depressed. A record called a pneumogram is obtained by allowing the stylus to write on a revolving drum which is covered by paper.

By attaching the pneumograph around the chest, the changes in the circumference of the chest will create length changes in the pneumograph. The resultant changes indicated by the writing stylus are proportional to the circumference (or volume) change in the individual. In speech application, the changes during various phonatory actions can be recorded.

In common electronic methods, circumference (volume) changes of the chest wall are detected by a special pneumograph containing a strain gauge which transduces the volume changes into electrical signals. The signals are amplified and are usually displayed on a strip chart recorder or a channel recorder. It is necessary that a staff member supervise the setting up of the apparatus.

PROCEDURE

Recording Human Respiratory Movements

The procedures below assume that mechanical pneumographs are being used.

1. Fasten the pneumograph around the chest of a student. Connect a piece of pressure tubing to one end. Attach a T-tube in series. The short limb of the T-tube is provided with a piece of rubber tubing which can be closed by a clamp. Connect the distal end of the T-tube with a Marey tambour. Add a signal magnet to your setup and connect it to a source arranged to give signals every second.

2. To obtain a good tracing, about an inch high, regulate the pressure in the tambour system by letting air into it or out of it through the T-tube. Close the T-tube after inflating the system. By the movements of the thorax, the air pressure in the tube of the pneumograph is altered; this is transmitted to the tambour. Note whether the lever rises or falls during inspiration. The subject must not look at the tracing, his attention being distracted by

reading. He is placed in comfortable sitting posture. Any alteration in the position or degree of inflation of the pneumograph will alter the amplitude of the lever; records cannot be compared under these conditions. The direction of inspiration or expiration should be indicated by an arrow.

3. Record 20 respiratory movements on a slow drum and 10 on a faster drum. Record time in seconds. Label. From your record: (1) calculate the rate of respiration; (2) measure the pause between inspiration and expiration in seconds, and between expiration and inspiration.

Abdominal vs. Costal Breathing

Place one pneumograph on the chest, and a second on the abdomen, to take simultaneous records. Line up the writing points. The leverages (amplitudes produced by a given change) upon the two tambours must be identical. Take records: (a) sitting and (b) standing. Compare the two kinds of breathing in the two positions. How does the rate compare in the two types in the two positions? How does the rate compare in the two types in any one position?

Effect of Speech Upon Breathing

Obtain a normal pneumogram, including several respiratory cycles. Read a paragraph or two from a text and analyze the effect of the speech upon the amplitude, rate and rhythm of the inspiratory and expiratory curves.

Repeat the reading, but whisper only. State any differences. Repeat the reading in a loud voice. State any differences.

Record the effect of laughing upon the respiratory rate, rhythm and amplitude. Then record the effect of singing.

Note on your records that during speaking the time relations of the phases of inhalation and exhalation are changed. Considerable time is spent in exhalation. There are less exhalations per minute and each inhalation is deeper. Exhalation becomes more forceful during speech.

Do not conclude that the rate of phonation is limited by the breathing mechanism. The muscles of breathing and speech are both regulated by control systems that may set similar upper limits (Wyke, 1974, p. 337).

REFERENCES

Exercise 11

Kaplan, H. M. **Anatomy and Physiology of Speech**. New York: McGraw-Hill Book Company, 1971.

McMinn, R. M. H. and Hutchings, R. T. **Color Atlas of Human Anatomy**. Chicago: Year Book Medical Publishers, 1977.

Minifie, R. D., Hixon, T. J. and Williams, F. (eds.). **Normal Aspects of Speech, Hearing and Language**. Englewood Cliffs, New Jersey: Prentice Hall, Inc., 1973.

Exercise 12

Dubois, A.B., Bothelho, S. Y. and Comroe, J. H. "A New Method of Measuring Airway Resistance in Man Using a Body Plethysmograph: Values in Normal Subjects and in Patients with Respiratory Disease." **Journal of Clinical Investigation**. 35:327-335, 1956.

Comroe, J. H. **Physiology of Respiration**. 2nd edition. Chicago: Year Book Medical Publishers, 1974.

Hixon T. J. and Warren, D. W. **Use of Plethysmographic Techniques in Speech Research: Two Laboratories Experiences**. Oral Presentation, American Speech and Hearing Association, Chicago, 1971.

Lass, N. J. (Ed.). **Contemporary Issues in Experimental Phonetics**. New York: Academic Press, 1976.

Wyke, B. (Ed.). **Ventilatory Phonatory Control Systems**. New York: Oxford University Press, 1974.

Exercise 13

Guyton, A. C. **Textbook of Medical Physiology**. 5th edition. Philadelphia: W. B. Saunders Company, 1976.

Kaplan, H. M. **Anatomy and Physiology of Speech**. 2nd edition. New York: McGraw-Hill Book Company, 1971.

Kaplan, H. M. and Spiegel, G. **The Physiology Laboratory**. Champaign, Ill.: Stipes Publishing Co., 1977.

Wyke, B. **Ventilatory and Phonatory Control Systems**. New York: Oxford University Press, 1974.

CHAPTER IV
Physics of Sound

EXERCISE 14

PROPERTIES OF WAVES

OBJECTIVES

Sound production involves complex waveforms. This brief Exercise is to introduce the student to the terminology and basic properties of waves. The procedures require supervision by a staff member familiar with oscilloscopes and basic electronic equipment. If necessary, the Exercise may be presented as a demonstration.

TIME REQUIRED

One laboratory period - two hours

MATERIALS

Microphones
Audioamplifiers
Oscilloscopes
Strip chart recorders

Sine wave oscillators or function
　　generators
Leads
Tuning forks

DESCRIPTION

Source of Sound Waves

Sound waves are produced by a vibrating body. In a simple system, with a tuning fork as the source, when the prongs move outward they compress the particles of the surrounding air and the compression is transmitted progressively outward by activation of the more peripheral particles. When the prongs reverse direction, the adjacent particles move back again producing a rarefaction. The alternate compressions and rarefactions in the air are expressed as longitudinal waves, the air particles being displaced along the axis of propagation of the wave. Vibrations which fall within the range of human hearing are called sound waves.

Terminology

If the pressure variations in air produced by a vibrating tuning fork are plotted against time, the curve is smooth with alternate peaks and troughs. This expresses the simplest waveform, called a sine wave, which exactly repeats itself (Figure 14-1). The tuning fork is unique in that it emits all its power in a simple sine wave at one frequency. Most other sources emit complex waves.

FIGURE 14-1
NATURE OF SINE WAVES

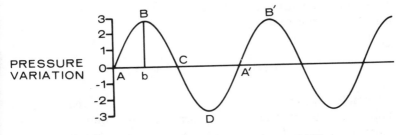

TIME, IN 0.01 SEC

In analyzing the sine wave of the tuning fork (Figure 14-1), the sequence of events represented by the line passing through ABCD'A is a cycle. The number of cycles per second is the frequency. The duration of time between any two equal points on successive waves is the period. The period (P) is the reciprocal of the frequency (f). If f is 256 Hz, P=1/256 seconds.

The maximum extent of the pressure change from the baseline is the amplitude, e.g. b to B. The amplitude quantitatively indicates the strength of the wave.

The wavelength (λ)is the distance between any two corresponding points in successive waves, e.g. B to'B. λ 's the velocity of sound in air, at a given temperature and frequency.

Complex Waves

If two tuning forks close to one another emit waves, one at 100 Hz and the other at 300, and both at different amplitudes, the compressions and rarefactions will mingle. The pressure is the resultant of the two original pressures and a complex wave having a unique, non-sinusoidal waveform results. This is only one example of a complex wave.

The original waves may have different starting points, say by 1/4 cycle. One wave reaches its maximum and minimum amplitudes 1/4 oscillation later than the other. This is a phase difference. If both waves were similar in period and amplitute and started simultaneously from the same source, a single wave would result and it would be the sum of the two waves. This is summation. It accounts for such biologic signals as the ECG, EEG and others. The ear does not use the phases of components to distinguish among complex waves, except perhaps to locate the direction of a source.

Analysis of Sound Waves

Complex waves can be broken down into their components. Fourier's theorem states that any periodic wave consists of one or more sine waves. Where the waves are exactly repetitive, the complex waveform is resolvable to a series of sinusoidal components and the frequencies of the components are integral multiples of the frequency of repetition of the original complex wave. The highest common factor of the component frequencies is the fundamental frequency, f_0. The sinusoidal components of such a waveform are harmonics.

Harmonic analysis is applicable only to periodic waves. At any point the total change of pressure with time in a complex wave is the algebraic sum of the changes produced by its individual components.

The ear can differentiate the sinusoidal components of the repetitive complex wave as pure tones of given amplitudes. This can be represented as a spectrum, plotting amplitude against frequency. This is a line spectrum showing the power of a sound wave, power being present only at certain frequencies (Figure 14-2). A continuous spectrum represents a sound wave whose power spreads over a range of frequencies, without periodicity. In Figure 14-2 the energy of two tuning forks is expressed only at specific frequencies.

PROCEDURE

I. Cathode Ray Oscilloscope: Waveform Visualization

An oscilloscope works by bombarding a phosphorescent screen with electrons in an evacuated tube with a filament as the electron source. The electrons excite the atoms in the screen and the energy is transduced to longer waves seen as visible light which persists. To prevent the electrons from burning a hole in the screen, the light is kept sweeping across the screen.

1. Turn on the oscilloscope. Note that a time control regulates the speed at which the beam sweeps across the screen. The control is usually calibrated in (sweep) time/cm and it tells the time for the beam to move 1 cm. A vertical control moves the beam up and down. An amplitude control in volts/cm regulates the vertical deflection (cm) for each volt or fraction of a volt originating from the source.
2. Adjust the scope to have a slow sweep and focus the beam.
3. Adjust each control to become familiar with the instrument.
4. Turn on a signal generator to produce sine waves and connect the generator to the oscilloscope. A sine wave should appear. If not, adjust the amplitude control to match the gain setting on the

FIGURE 14-2
LINE SPECTRUM

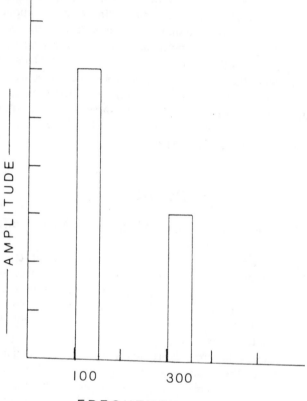

FREQUENCY (Hz)

oscilloscope or vice versa. If you cannot get a signal, the signal and ground leads may be reversed.

5. On some oscilloscopes, the sweep can be triggered by several modes. Internal triggering will suffice here.

6. Manipulate the generator to increase the frequency of the sine waves. A greater number of waves will be seen in a given time. Reducing the frequency decreases the rate of production of waves.

Note that increasing the frequency decreases the period of the sine wave.

7. Set up a strip chart recorder and connect the signal generator to it instead of to the oscilloscope. A record of the waveforms can then be obtained with penwriters. The chart should have a zero control for positioning the pen, a speed control to set the paper speed, a lever for putting the pen on the paper, and perhaps an amplitude control. Adjust the pen to the middle of the paper. Set the generator to 10 Hz and turn on the paper drive and signal generator. The paper should be moving and the pen oscillating. Obtain a record. If the pen strikes limits of range, decrease the input amplitude.

8. Vary the input signal frequency from the generator. Observe the changes on the record in frequency and period of the waves.

II. Oscilloscope: Wave Summation

1. Connect the signal generator to the oscilloscope and set the time base to a sweep that will display two waves for a 10 Hz input signal. Adjust the amplitude to give a peak to peak deflection of 2 cm. Set a second generator at 10 Hz with an identical amplitude setting and connect it to the same oscilloscope. By matching the frequency settings on the two oscillators, you should get a single sine wave. From Figure 14-3, draw simultaneous waves A and B as a single, complex wave in C.

2. Change the frequency of one generator to exactly twice the frequency of the other. Note the change in the waveform.

3. Add a third generator at three times the frequency of the slowest wave. What name applies to the lowest frequency and the other two waves?

III. Demonstration of a Complex Wave

1. Set up a audioamplifier (and be sure a speaker is connected to prevent burning out the output transformer). Connect a microphone to the amplifier and connect the amplifier output to the oscilloscope. Check the amplitude of the amplifier to match the amplitude of the oscilloscope. Set the oscilloscope beam to a moderate

FIGURE 14-3
SUMMATION OF WAVES

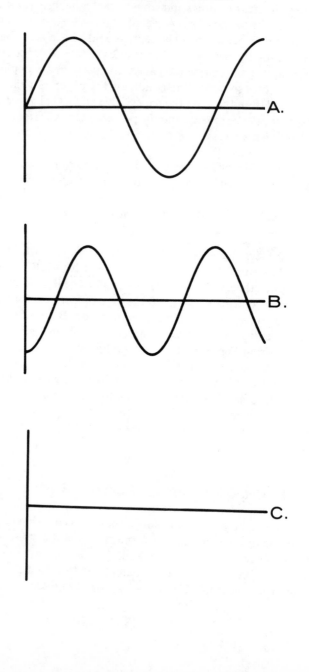

speed.

2. Turn on the audioamplifier and speak into the microphone. Observe complex waveforms on the oscilloscope screen.

3. Sound a tuning fork which puts a pure tone into the microphone. Note the form of the wave.

4. Select vowels and pronounce them successively into the microphone. Do this softly, then loudly. Note the waveforms.

5. Phonate several consonants into the microphone and observe the characteristic pattern of each sound. If clear differences are not noticeable, try adjusting the amplitude or frequency of the sweep.

6. These sounds may be recorded on the strip chart recorder to produce spectrograms. Explain the possibilities of spectrograms for the analysis of speech.

7. What is the relationship of sine waves and Fourier Analysis to speech spectrograms?

REVIEW

1. Define: amplitude, period, frequency, phase difference or phase angle, simple harmonic action, summation, sinusoidal wave, fundamental, harmonic, Fourier analysis.

2. Explain how the waves are summated in Figure 14-3.

REFERENCES

Exercise 14

Barber, N. F. **Experimental Correlograms and Fourier Transforms.** New York: Pergamon Press, 1961.

Bouhuys, A. (Ed.). **Sound Production in Man.** Annals of the New York Academy of Sciences, Volume 155, Article 1, 1968.

Brosnahan, L. F. and Malmberg, B. **Introduction to Phonetics.** Cambridge, England: W. Heffer and Sons Ltd., 1970.

CHAPTER V
Larynx and Phonation

EXERCISE 15

HUMAN LARYNGEAL ANATOMY

OBJECTIVES

Larynges can be made available from human cadavers. We do this by arrangement with our medical school and recommend such liaisons wherever possible. Dissection of the excised larynx can be performed in accordance with the directions herein under supervision of a staff member familiar with anatomic dissection procedures. It is possible in the isolated larynx to visualize the cartilage framework, connecting membranes, nerves and arrangement of the musculature. The student must take great care first to observe and only then to dissect. Precise dissection is a highly disciplined procedure, but a rewarding one as well as evaluative of the student's manual dexterity.

TIME REQUIRED

One to two laboratory periods - two to four hours depending partly upon supervisory expertise.

MATERIALS

Excised and preserved human larynges, with hyoid bone and all muscles attached (Commercially obtained sheep larynges may be substituted if human larynges cannot be made available)

Scalpels, blades, scissors, forceps and probes
Dissection pans
Charts and models of the larynx
Atlas and dissection manual (see References)

DESCRIPTION AND PROCEDURE

Before dissecting the preserved wet specimens, examine in detail models and charts of the larynx. Then try to locate and identify the structures described herein. Each group should be provided with two or more preserved larynges.

The endings of nerves should have been left intact when the anatomy prosector removed the larynx from the cadaver. Examine the isolated larynx for the presence of these nerves before proceeding to any dissection.

The recurrent (inferior) laryngeal nerve arises from the main vagal trunk below the larynx and ascends on each side in a groove between the trachea and esophagus. The nerve divides at the inferior border of the cricoid. The posterior branch supplies the posterior cricoarytenoid and the oblique and transverse arytenoid muscles. The anterior branch supplies the lateral cricoarytenoid, thyroarytenoid and vocalis muscles. The recurrent nerve supplies all muscles of the larynx except the cricothyroid.

The superior laryngeal nerve leaves the main vagal trunk at the upper level of the thyroid cartilage and crosses medially to enter the thyrohyoid membrane. This nerve innervates the cricothyroid muscle and it also provides the major sensory supply of the larynx.

EXTERNAL LANDMARKS (FIGURES 15-1 AND 15-2)

Palpate the larynx in all its external aspects to find its regional cartilaginous structures. Locate the laryngeal prominence and thyroid notch. Feel the superior and inferior cornua of the thyroid cartilage.

FIGURE 15-1
ANTERIOR VIEW OF CARTILAGES OF LARYNX

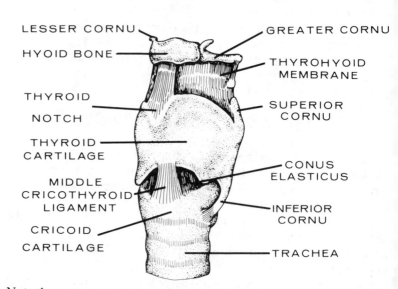

Note the extent of the thyroid lamina. Locate the cricoid cartilage just below the thyroid cartilage. Follow the cricoid ring posteriorly to find the enlarged signet-like cricoid lamina. Hold the epiglottis firmly and follow the aryepiglottic fold down to the midline posteriorly, feeling gently for the cuneiform and corniculate cartilages. Having located the laryngeal cartilages, palpate the hyoid bone and its cornua.

Folds, Membranes and Ligaments (Figures 15-1 and 15-3)

Connective tissue in the form of membranes fills in the gaps between the cartilages. Connective tissue also forms the framework of both the true and false folds. Examine both the exterior and interior of the larynx to locate the following membranes and ligaments.

The thyrohyoid membrane is attached superiorly to the body and cornua of the hyoid bone. It is attached inferiorly to the superior cornua and superior borders of the thyroid cartilage laminae. It is best seen in the anterior view of the larynx.

FIGURE 15-2

SAGITTAL SECTION OF HEAD SHOWING PHARYNX AND GENERAL RELATIONSHIPS OF LARYNX

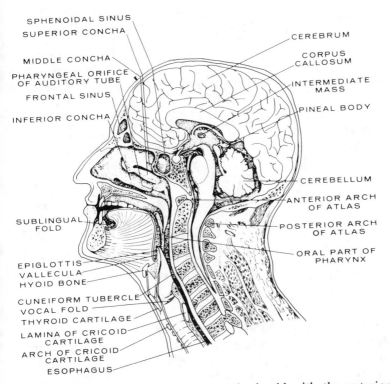

The hyoepiglottic ligament connects the hyoid with the anterior aspect of the epiglottis.

The thyroepiglottic ligament connects the epiglottis to the thyroid cartilage.

The cricotracheal ligament connects the inferior border of the cricoid to the uppermost tracheal cartilage.

The cricothyroid ligament is located in the midline anteriorly, extending up from the cricoid arch in a fan-shaped manner to the inferior border of the thyroid cartilage.

The lateral segments of the cricothyroid ligament on each side extend up and under the thyroid laminae. At their upper edges they merge into the conus elasticus (on each side). These connective tissues

FIGURE 15-3
POSTERIOR VIEW OF CARTILAGES OF LARYNX

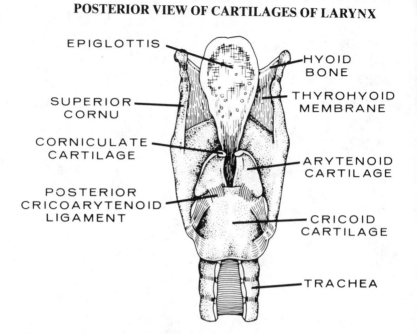

extend superiorly and their upper free borders form the vocal ligament, or platform of the true vocal folds. In the horizontal plane the vocal ligaments stretch on each side from the thyroid angle anteriorly to the vocal processes of the arytenoids posteriorly.

The quadrangular membrane extends downward from the posterolateral aspects of the epiglottis and it ends on each side in free borders which form the vestibular ligaments, or platforms for the paired false vocal folds.

Cartilages (Figures 15-1 and 15-3)

Using laryngeal models and charts, conceptualize the structure and relationships of the cartilage framework. Then proceed to the dissection of the specimen. Try to locate all structures described herein.

Epiglottis

This is the highest cartilage. It is leaf-shaped. Its stem attaches by a thyroepiglottic ligament to the inner aspect of the thyroid cartilage just below the thyroid notch. Examine the coverings of the epiglottis. The coverings include mucous membrane and glossoepiglottic folds (one medial and two lateral). These folds pass between the epiglottis and the tongue, leaving between the two structures depressions called valleculae.

Thyroid Cartilage

This single structure is the largest cartilage of the larynx and it is formed by two anterolateral plates (laminae) that are fused in the midline anteriorly but divergent posteriorly. Projections from the posterior edges extend superiorly as the superior horns and inferiorly as the inferior horns (cornua). The anterosuperior area of union of the plates presents a midline thyroid notch.

Cricoid Cartilage

This single structure forms the lower skeleton of the larynx and it is the only complete ring in the airway. Its posterior part is enlarged to a signet-like lamina while its anterior extensions are curved into a ring-like arch. The superior border of the signet has a pair of facets for articulation with the arytenoid cartilages.

Arytenoid Cartilages

These paired structures are relatively small. They articulate with the cricoid cartilages such that gliding and rocking motions can occur. Each pyramidal-shaped arytenoid cartilage presents three surfaces. The vocal processes at the anteromedial base of each arytenoid provides attachment for the vocal ligament (skeleton of the true vocal folds). Muscular processes at the posterolateral base allow insertion of several intrinsic muscles which move the arytenoid cartilages.

Corniculate Cartilages

These are two small paired nodules, each of which caps the apex of an arytenoid cartilage. Their functions are obscure.

Cuneiform Cartilages

These are small paired nodules, each imbedded in an aryepiglottic fold (which stretches from each side of the epiglottis down to the corresponding arytenoid).

Joints

There are two paired joints of major importance, both freely movable and both permitting rotary and gliding movements. These are the cricothyroid joints and cricoarytenoid joints. They should be manipulated on models and also on the specimen to visualize their movements.

Muscles (Superficial; Figures 15-4 and 15-5)

Identify muscles first in models and charts and then in the isolated specimen. By cleaning the overlying fascia, locate each cricothyroid muscle running from the anterolateral section of the cricoid arch up and back to each inferior cornu of the thyroid cartilage.

Clean away the fascia on the posterior aspect of the specimens and locate the posterior cricoarytenoid, oblique arytenoid and transverse arytenoid muscles.

The posterior cricoarytenoid muscle originates on each side from the posterior part of the cricoid. It passes superolaterally to insert on the muscular process of the arytenoid.

Observe posteriorly the superficial oblique arytenoid and the deeper transverse arytenoid muscles filling the concavities of the arytenoid cartilages. The oblique fibers originate from the muscular process of the arytenoid and travel superomedially to insert on the apex of the arytenoid of the other side. Extensions superiorly of these fibers to the

FIGURE 15-4
LATERAL VIEW OF MUSCLES OF LARYNX

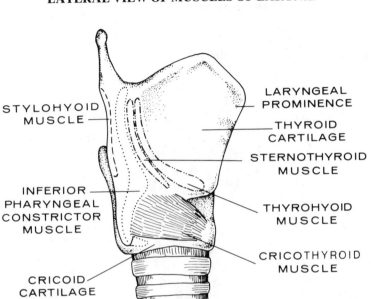

epiglottis form the paired aryepiglottic muscles. The single transverse arytenoid muscle originates on the posterior aspect of one arytenoid, crosses the median line, and inserts on the posterior aspect of the opposite arytenoid cartilage.

Turn to the anterior aspect of the larynx. Locate the paired, ribbon-like sternohyoid and sternothyroid muscles. Place a finger on the laryngeal prominence and move it laterally along the lamina. A small muscle, the thyrohyoid muscle, will be encountered. The thyrohyoid, sternothyroid, and inferior pharyngeal constrictor muscles all attach to the thyroid cartilage along an oblique line on the lamina. Distinguish each muscle as well as the cricothyroid which attaches directly below the common attachment.

Muscles (Internal; Figure 15-6)

To get to the deeper muscles it is necessary to dissect away structures. If this is done only on one side of the specimen, structures to be

FIGURE 15-5
POSTERIOR VIEW OF MUSCLE S OF LARYNX

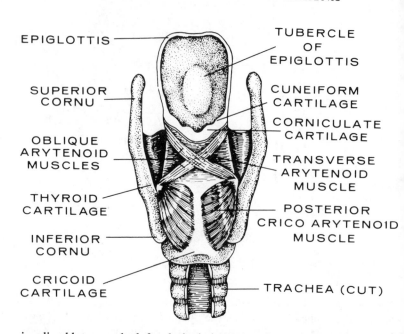

EPIGLOTTIS

TUBERCLE OF EPIGLOTTIS

SUPERIOR CORNU

CUNEIFORM CARTILAGE

CORNICULATE CARTILAGE

OBLIQUE ARYTENOID MUSCLES

TRANSVERSE ARYTENOID MUSCLE

THYROID CARTILAGE

POSTERIOR CRICO ARYTENOID MUSCLE

INFERIOR CORNU

CRICOID CARTILAGE

TRACHEA (CUT)

visualized later can be left relatively intact on the opposite side.

Reflect the muscles attached to the lamina on one side of the thyroid cartilage. Transect the thyrohyoid membrane holding that side of the thyroid cartilage and hyoid bone. Free the posterior two-thirds of the inside of the exposed thyroid lamina. Transect the cricothyroid membrane binding the cricoid and thyroid cartilages. Dissect the fascia from the exposed internal regions deep to the thyroid laminae. You should now see the lateral cricoarytenoid, aryepiglottic, thyroepiglottic, thyroarytenoid and vocalis muscles.

The paired lateral cricoarytenoid muscles lie on the cricoid arch just within each thyroid lamina. The muscles originate from the anterolateral aspects of the cricoid arch, travel posterosuperiorly, and insert on the muscular processes of the arytenoid cartilages.

The paired thyroarytenoid muscles originate posterior (internal) to the union (angle) of the laminae of the thyroid cartilage. The throarytenoid fibers travel posteriorly and insert on the muscular

FIGURE 15-6
LATERAL VIEW OF INTRINSIC MUSCLES
OF LARYNX

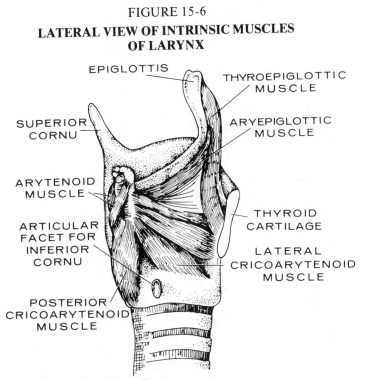

processes of the arytenoid cartilages.

The vocalis muscles form much of the flesh of the vocal folds. They originate in the same location as that of the thyroarytenoid muscles. The vocalis muscles extend posteriorly and insert on the vocal processes of the arytenoid cartilages.

The aryepiglottic and thyroepiglottic muscles need not be followed in detail.

Laryngeal Cavities (Figures 15-7 and 15-8)

Observe on charts and models that the great cavity of the laryngeal interior may be arbitrarily divided to three compartments. Note on the isolated specimen that the uppermost compartment, or vestibule, extends down from the inlet to the false (ventricular) vocal folds. The middle compartment, or ventricle, extends down from the ventricular

FIGURE 15-7
CORONAL SECTION OF LARYNX

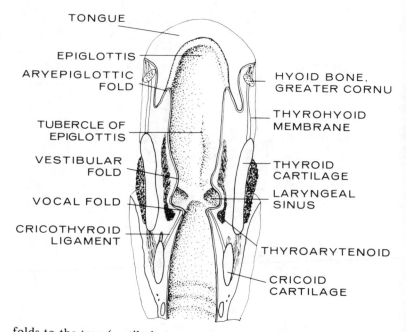

TONGUE

EPIGLOTTIS

ARYEPIGLOTTIC
FOLD

HYOID BONE,
GREATER CORNU

THYROHYOID
MEMBRANE

TUBERCLE OF
EPIGLOTTIS

VESTIBULAR
FOLD

THYROID
CARTILAGE

LARYNGEAL
SINUS

VOCAL FOLD

CRICOTHYROID
LIGAMENT

THYROARYTENOID

CRICOID
CARTILAGE

folds to the true (vestibular) vocal folds. The space between the true folds is the glottis (rima glottidis). The lowest compartment is the inferior division, or atrium. It descends from the true folds to the first tracheal cartilage.

EXERCISE 16

OBSERVATION OF THE HUMAN LARYNX
BY INDIRECT LARYNGOSCOPY

OBJECTIVES

The student can visualize the larynx by this procedure both in struc-

FIGURE 15-8
SAGITTAL SECTION OF LARYNX

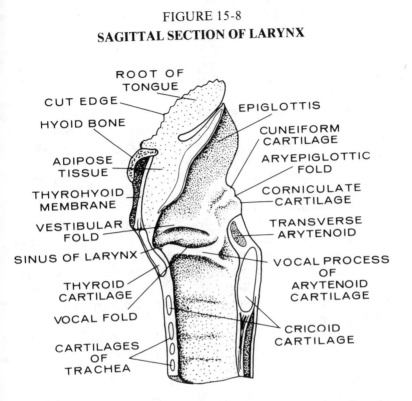

ture and action. He can within the limits of his experience translate the appearance of the previously dissected larynx to its behavior in life. All students in each group should examine the larynx of one another.

TIME REQUIRED

Two hours if each individual participates

MATERIALS

Electric head lamps, or else light source (150 watt lamp) and head mirrors

Laryngeal mirrors
Gauze squares or tongue depressors

DESCRIPTION AND PROCEDURE

The beginner must not try to perform this Exercise without assistance. Although this is essentially a non-invasive activity, since only a laryngeal mirror enters the fauces, expert instructional guidance should be available.

Adequate illumination is necessary and it may be provided either by transmitting light into the throat from an electric head lamp, or by directing light from a light bulb onto a clinical head mirror which then transmits the beam into the throat. The examiner must focus the light accurately, since correct alignment of the light reflection from the laryngeal mirror is needed to assure proper illumination of the interior of the larynx (Figure 16-1).

The image seen in the laryngeal mirror which is at the fauces (passage between mouth and throat) is the reflected one, which is reversed in the anteroposterior plane but true in the lateral plane. Some foreshortening of the image in the anteroposterior plane also results from the use of the mirror. From the examiner's position, facing the subject, the subject's right vocal fold is on the examiner's left side. Because of image reversal, the anterior commissure of the larynx seems to the examiner to be directly posteriorly. The instructor can simplify the beginner's confusion by likening the glottis to a capital A, remembering that in the open glottis the apex points anteriorly.

The subject must be sitting upright, on the same level as that of the examiner, with the head drawn a little forward. The choice of laryngeal mirror size is important since too large a mirror could produce a gag relex if it hit certain mucosal receptors and one that is too small could be extended behind the palate.

With the subject's tongue extended, a sterile gauze square is wrapped around the tongue tip to protect the undersurface and the frenulum of the tongue from the lower teeth. The examiner holds the gauze-wrapped tongue with the first and third fingers of his left hand and uses his index finger to elevate the upper lip. The mirror is warmed slightly, its temperature is tested on the dorsum of the hand, and it is inserted slowly into the mouth, care being taken to avoid touching the tongue. While the subject breathes quickly, the mirror is placed against the uvula, pushing it upward and backward. The examiner's light on his forehead is focused on the laryngeal mirror, the latter then being tilted at various angles to obtain a good reflected image of the larynx.

FIGURE 16-1
INDIRECT LARYNGOSCOPY

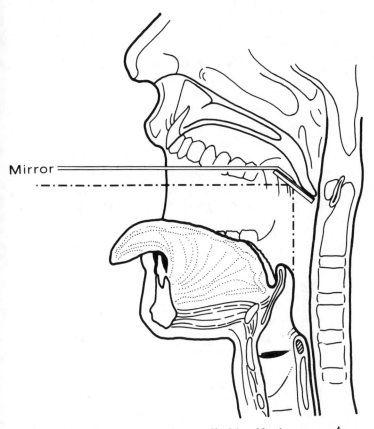

Mirror

The student is not expected to easily identify the structures coming into view and the following may be pointed out. When the laryngeal mirror is introduced, the first structure seen is the back of the tongue with its large follicles, then the hollow space between it and the dark-pink, glossal (anterior) surface of the epiglottis. The apex and laryngeal surface of the epiglottis are next seen, the free surface being yellowish and the laryngeal (under surface) bright red. The aryepiglottic folds have about the same color as the mucous membrane of the gums. The ventricular folds have about the same color as the mucous lining of the lips. The true vocal folds are pearly white, like the sclerotic (outer) coat of the eye. Visualize the tracheal ring outlines which are yellow, the mucous membrane between them being bright red.

When the dorsal wall of the larynx is brought into view, observe the form, size, color, position, and mobility of the true and false vocal folds.

An instructor with clinical experience can point out indications of pathology. The mucous membrane may appear red, swollen, or ulcerated. The vocal folds may be pale or red, display ecchymotic spots, or be covered by a thick stringy secretion.

To obtain a wider velopharyngeal port so as to better visualize the larynx, ask the subject to produce and sustain the vowel sound /E/ as in sEt or /i:/ as in bEEt. These sounds are associated with elevation of the velum. If the subject produces an /a/ sound as in ah, the tongue is depressed which also permits widening of the faucial port.

Sketch what you have seen in the "resting" phases and in phonating other vowels. How does pitch change affect the nature of the valving?

EXERCISE 17

ANALYSIS OF HUMAN MUSCLE ACTIVITY BY ELECTROMYOGRAPHY

OBJECTIVES

This Exercise should acquaint the student with a basic electromyographic procedure for visualizing action potentials from living muscles in action.

Action potentials are to be studied from the conveniently located biceps muscle of the arm during isotonic and isometric exercise. Although the biceps has no relation to laryngeal or oral function, its study brings out the general principles of methodology which the student should learn. If time permits, extrinsic muscles of the larynx can be similarly examined. Supervision by a staff member is necessary and a demonstration prior to student participation is recommended.

TIME REQUIRED

One laboratory period - two hours

MATERIALS

Channel recorders or electromyographs (containing cathode
ray oscilloscope display)
Leads
Surface electrodes (floating or disposable

Electrode paste
70 per cent ethyl alcohol
15 and 25 pound weights

DESCRIPTION

Equipment

The student needs to know some general facts about the equipment he is asked to use since the specific equipment importantly determines the validity of the data obtained.

Unlike ECG and EEG recording, the electromyograph (EMG) requires a higher frequency response. Pen recorders do not follow high frequency signals. The readout for the EMG is thus accomplished by a cathode ray oscilloscope placed into the circuit. Although it is ordinarily best not to utilize the pen-writers which are found on channel recorders, this is feasible, nevertheless, in student work where the emphasis is on general facts and principles. It is to be recognized, however, that faithful response and exact quantitation will not be achieved.

Commercial electromyographs (Hewlett-Packard Co., Waltham, Mass., or other vendors) may include an audioamplifier and loudspeaker so that characteristic sounds can be heard which help the operator to place electrodes correctly on a muscle.

Electromyograph amplifiers should have high gain and high input impedance. The muscle potentials produce a noiselike waveform varying in amplitude with changes in muscle activity. Peak amplitudes vary from 50 microvolts to about one millivolt. The frequency response varies from 10 to more than 3,000 Hz.

Electrodes are of several types. Surface electrodes have a limited usefulness. They may be used where muscles are close to the cutaneous surface and penetration of the skin is undesirable. They tend to produce only small potentials which are susceptible to interference. They are useful in student laboratories because they are non-invasive and still capable of producing data which illustrate basic principles.

Intramuscular electrodes provide increased precision and specificity. The most common is the concentric needle electrode which is a hypodermic needle with an insulated wire fixed in the cannula. There is also a hooked-wire electrode, commonly used, which has two fine insulated wires threaded through a hypodermic needle and bent to the shape of a hook. The guilding hypodermic needle is removed from the overlying skin, leaving the hooked wires implanted into the muscle. The flexibility of the wires minimizes body movement artifacts.

For student work neither the coaxial electrode in which a wire is inside a hypodermic needle nor the bipolar electrode consisting of two wires is recommended. This dictum is stated despite the fact that intramuscular electrodes may be thin, relatively painless, easily implanted and productive of sharp spike potentials. Implantation takes experience and cautious supervision.

In using surface electrodes, attach them to the skin over selected motor points of the biceps muscle of the dominant arm. Small "floating" electrodes are adequate in localizing the potentials. Prior to placement, shave the area and clean it with 70 per cent ethyl alcohol. Fill the floating electrodes with electrode paste and bring them close to the skin by double adhesive discs straddling the motor points and parallel with the long axis of the muscle. Place the ground electrode over a nearby area where there are few muscles, such as the wrist or sternum.

Theory

Contraction of muscle is accompanied by electrochemical changes expressed as action potentials. The recording of action potentials in active muscles is the basis of electromyography. The procedure is founded on observations that resting muscle is isopotential and generates no current. When a muscle is stimulated, the resulting excitation travels along the muscle as waves of action potential. If two electrodes are attached to the skin over the muscle, they can pick up the potentials. Since each motor unit (nerve fiber and the muscle fibers it supplies) responds repetitively during activity, the electrodes pick up the electric potentials of all the motor units within the recording range.

PROCEDURE

1. Calibrate the equipment. This varies with different channel recorders and electromyographs. In using a channel recorder, set the paper speed at about 25 mm/second.
2. If there is considerable noise in the signal from the subject's biceps area, suspect high electrical resistance of the skin. It may be necessary to remove the electrodes and paste and re-prepare the skin surface.
3. After the skin electrodes have been connected and a calibration signal has been obtained, have the subject stand and perform an isometric contraction in which he or she holds a 15-lb weight in a semiflexed position with the dominant arm for one minute. Simultaneously obtain EMG records on channel recorders (or note the calibrated deflections on the oscilloscope). The subject is to follow this immediately by the same type of exercise with the dominant arm for one more minute with a 25-lb weight. Again obtain EMG records during the isometric contraction.
4. Give the subject a 15-lb weight and have him or her commence isotonic elbow flexion curls with the nondominant arm for one minute. The subject is to follow this by one minute of the same exercise with a 25-lb weight. Obtain EMG records for both bouts of isotonic exercise.
5. Allow rest periods (5 min.) between isometric and isotonic exercises.
6. For each exercise, mark 10 second time intervals on the records and record the peak deflections (amplitudes) in mm produced by the muscle. Derive action potential values from each exercise by averaging the peak deflections from all of the 10 speed time measures and expressing them in microvoltage.
7. Present the data in tabular form.

EXERCISE 18

FACTORS INFLUENCING RESPIRATION
AND LARYNGEAL MOVEMENTS

OBJECTIVES

The student can gain some facility in conducting an experiment with a living (anesthetized) animal (rabbit) and can visualize directly structure in action.

Supervision by a staff member is essential. Each student group should have continual access to assistants who have had experience particularly with animal anesthesia and euthanasia. This experiment can be performed as a demonstration.

TIME REQUIRED

One laboratory period - three hours

MATERIALS

Ether
Nose cones and gauze
Tracheal cannulas
Pneumographs
Marey tambours
Pressure tubing
Surgical instruments
Heart levers
Pulleys
Electronic stimulators

Kymographs or channel recorders
Animal clippers
Bottle with two hole stoppers to
    allow air entrance at one end
    which mixes with ether in the
    bottle, the anesthetic mixture
    coming out at the end connected
    to the tracheal cannual
White New Zealand rabbit, 2 to
    3 kg. body weight.

DESCRIPTION AND PROCEDURE

Although this exercise emphasizes selected respiratory as well as laryngeal phenomena, the latter has a special interest. The student should review laryngeal anatomy in the human prior to undertaking the surgical procedure.

FACTORS INFLUENCING BREATHING

Etherize a rabbit and expose the caudal part of the trachea, avoiding the more cranial pharyngeal and hyoid regions.

Make a double T-shaped incision in the trachea, the long arms pointing toward the lungs in the lower opening and connect it by a cannula with the ether bottle as needed. In the upper opening insert a cannula pointed toward the nasal cavities.

Expose both vagus nerves in the ventral neck and place loose lifting ligatures under them. Arrange to record breathing. In laboratories using manual equipment (all obtainable from Harvard Apparatus Co., Millis, MA. 02054), rotate a kymograph drum just quickly enough to resolve individual respiratory cycles. Use either a thread passing from a pin, placed in the xiphoid skin of the rabbit, to a pulley system and then to a heart lever, or else use a small animal pneumograph tied around the rabbit's chest and connected by pressure tubing to a Marey tambour whose lever writes on the moving drum.

For the newer and more preferable electronic channel recorders (e.g. Physiograph system, Narco Bio-Systems, Houston, Texas 77017), impedance pneumographs and bellows type pneumographs are available.

The impedance pneumograph is a transducer/preamplifier for the quantitative measurement of respiratory rates and relative volumes and flow patterns in man and animals. Two needles, or two disc or plate electrodes are attached to the rabbit. A small alternating current is passed through the electrodes. The voltage across the electrodes is directly proportional to the rabbit's impedance. Voltage changes because of impedance changes are amplified for pen recording on a channel recorder. (We use an impedance pneumograph with the Physiograph.)

The alternative bellows-type pneumograph is a photoelectric transducer that works much like a (muscle) myograph, but it is specialized to record thoracic respiratory movements. We use the Narco Bio-Systems pneumograph. This consists of a negative pressure transducer with an attached flexible neoprene bellows and an adjustable strap to keep the bellows firmly adherent to the moving chest wall. The instrument shows rates, time sequences, and patterns of movement when the recording is seen on a channel recorder, e.g. Physiograph.

Data Collection

Obtain a short record; then lighten the anesthesia as judged by relexes and movements and obtain another strip of respiratory cycles. Etherize deeply through the bottle connected to the lower cannula and observe the effect upon respiration.

Lighten the anesthesia and obtain a record. Then place an ether cone over the nose of the animal and suck ether through the nasal cavities by aspiration through the upper tracheal cannula. Record the effects on the moving paper.

Deeply anesthetize the animal through the lower cannula. Then suck in ether through the nasal cone by aspiration through the upper cannula. Record the effects.

While the rabbit is under deep anesthesia, cut both vagus nerves low in the neck, and allow recovery from the anesthesia. Again aspirate ether through the nasal cone and observe the record.

Summarize the influence of ether upon respiratory reflexes as follows: (a) nasal reflex effects; (b) deep lung reflexes; and (c) the path of the reflexes as shown by the experimental evidence.

Factors Influencing Laryngeal Movements

Extend the upper tracheal incision cranially, avoiding the superficial blood vessels, which should be tied and reflected with the skin. Expose the thyroid and cricoid cartilages.

Isolate the upper continuation of the vagus nerves and find the superior laryngeal branch on one side. This is given off at the level of origin of the internal carotid artery. It crosses the dorsal side of the common carotid artery to reach the larynx, where it gives sensory fibers to the mucous membrane and motor fibers to the cricothyroid muscle.

Expose the cranial opening of the larynx by cutting transversely across the pharynx between the hyoid bone and the thyroid cartilage. Bring the tip of the epiglottis through the incision and secure it with a hemostat. Enlarge the cut laterally to raise the larynx and examine its internal aspect.

Data Collection

Identify the glottis and the rudimentary vocal folds. Note the changes in the glottis during quiet respiration, and then make the changes more conspicuous by closing the lower tracheal cannula to produce dyspnea.

Obtain records of all the following procedures. Stimulate the laryngeal mucosa with absorbent cotton and observe inhibition of respiration and forced expiration (coughing).

Stimulate the superior laryngeal nerve with weak faradic current from a stimulator and record the effects upon respiration and laryngeal movements.

Cut the superior laryngeal nerve between two ligatures, stimulate its distal and then its central end, and record the effects in each instance.

The laryngeal musculature, except for the cricothyroid, is supplied by the inferior laryngeal nerve and a search for the latter should be made at the inferior aspect of the larynx. Stimulate this nerve with faradic shocks and record its effects upon respiratory movements and upon the action of the laryngeal muscles. Cut the nerve between two ligatures, stimulate its distal and then its central end and analyze the effects in each instance.

This is an "acute" procedure. Euthanatize the rabbit with an overdose of the anesthetic used.

EXERCISE 19

PHONATION IN THE HUMAN LARYNX

OBJECTIVES

The student should observe external, gross laryngeal movements during phonation in the living person along with the nature of the associated breath support. The functional parameters of pitch and loudness should also be roughly evaluated. This Exercise relates to the mechanisms considered in Exercises 15 and 16 and the latter two should be reviewed. The observations involved should acquaint the student with some limited problems of the larynx in action.

TIME REQUIRED

One laboratory period - two hours

MATERIAL

Volume-level or sound-level meter

DESCRIPTION AND PROCEDURE

Palpation of Laryngeal Skeleton

Inspection and palpation are standard procedures in physical examination. By applying light pressure, locate on the human neck the hyoid bone, the upper and lower borders of the thyroid cartilage, cricoid cartilage, and trachea. Which of these structures are visible by external inspection?

Maintain the palpation and try to sense any movement or relation among the structural parts in the following actions:

        Breathing through the mouth
        Breathing through the nose
        Swallowing

CHEWING MOVEMENTS
Vocalizing Vowel Phonemes

Unwanted Movements During Phonation

A quick general assessment of voice can be made by seeing and hearing. Note while your laboratory partner is speaking in a conversational voice any evidence of high tension. For example, does the thyroid cartilage become quite elevated? Do the neck muscles appear to contract strongly? Use other members of the group for comparison. Is the pitch range appropriate to sex and age? Are there noises which may indicate faulty involvement of the false folds or other supraglottic structures? Does unvocalized breath escape? Is the loudness relatively strong or weak? Is the voice lacking in variety? Are the rate and rhythm of speaking normal? Undertake each of the above observations separately.

Voiced and Voiceless Consonants

The following tests show a difference between voiced and voiceless consonants. The former distinctly involve glottic activity.

Close both ears with the fingers and pronounce successively /f/ and /v/, /s/ and /z/, /f/ and /z/. Note the increased sensation of vibration in the ears for the voiced sounds. This expresses the emphasis of the bone conduction element of autofeedback. Similar tests can be made with other pairs, but with less distinction since each sound in these pairs may be so brief in isolation that it is difficult to obtain a satisfactory impression of the sound.

Place the hand against the throat with the crotch of the thumb and forefinger astride the larynx and pronounce /f,v/, /s,z/ and /f,z/. Note the sensation of vibration with the voiced sounds.

Adequacy of Exhalation for Phonation

Have the subject maximally inhale and then sustain a hissing, non-vocalized s-s-s, as long as possible. The average time for an adult is 20 seconds. This measures the sustained exhalation time independently of phonation. The sustained voiced exhalation for z-z-z should also be about 20 seconds. Subjects with vocal fold thickening, nodules, or polyps tend to perform well on the voiceless s-s-s, but usually will not prolong the voiced z-z-z.

General Aspects of Breath Support in Phonation

Have the subject read a passage of prose. Does the speaker produce a gasp at the close of a phrase or group of phrases? This suggests a faulty breath supply, but does not indicate the cause.

Does the speaker appear to exert excessive effort, drawing on his expiratory reserve volume? This suggests inadequate tidal volume.

Does the speaker exhale most of his breath supply prior to the start of speaking, heard as disruptions of phrasing and insufficient intensity of voice?

Does the speaker waste the air, indicating a breathy voice which may be wavering and tremorous?

Observe each action in succession. Use several subjects.

Phonation Time

Standing with normal posture, have the subject prolong the vowel /O/ as in nOtation at medium pitch and intensity for as long as possible, without preparatory deep inhalation. From five trials compute an average phonation time. The phonation time should average 15 to 20 seconds per breath.

Repeat the experiment, in the standing position, for other phonemes, determining the length of time that the subject can sustain each, but this time after deep inspiration.

Phonation and Optimum Vocal Frequency

For the speaking voice, several procedures have been proposed for estimating the natural, or optimum vocal frequency (optimum pitch). There are serious objections to many of these claims, including the one described below which is included only as an illustrative rule-of-thumb procedure. In this method, described by Hamlet et. al. (1973), sing down to the lowest note that you can sing. Do not make it so low that it sounds like choking or growling. Then sing up four notes (do-re-mi-fa). The fa is claimed to be a very rough approximation of the optimum frequency. Among other objections, this method fails to consider the view that the appropriate pitch is a range and not a specific tone or frequency.

Phonation and Pitch Stability

Ask the speaker to prolong the vowel/a/ as in fAther at a comfortable pitch level as long and as steadily as he can. A pronounced vocal tremor could suggest neurologic involvement at some level of the central nervous system. This conclusion would have to be correlated with other clinical data. Some tremors are psychogenic.

Phonation and Loudness Level

Optimal loudness is a quality of voice that is appropriate to the circumstance. Measure the loudness level of conversational speech of your partners with a volume-level meter or a sound-level meter. Loudness deviations occur in several disorders, e.g. cerebral palsy, Parkinson's disease, breathy voice, and others.

The examination of phonation should cover pitch, loudness and quality, separately and in combination. Since all three involve the vocal folds, their disorders can be associated with each other (Darley, 1964).

REFERENCES

Exercise 15

Anderson, J. E. **Grant's Atlas of Anatomy.** 7th edition. Baltimore: The Williams and Wilkins Company, 1976.

Fink, B. R. **The Human Larynx: A Functional Study.** New York: Raven Press, 1975.

McMinn, R. W. H. and Hutchings, R. T. **Color Atlas of Human Anatomy.** Chicago: Year Book Publishing Company, 1977.

Tobin, C. E. **Shearer's Manual of Human dissection.** 5th edition. New York: McGraw-Hill Book Company, 1967.

Warwick, R. and Williams, P. L. **Gray's Anatomy.** 6th edition. Philadelphia: W. B. Saunders Company, 1980.

Exercise 16

Paparella, M. M. and Shumrich, D. A. (Eds.). **Otolaryngology.** Volume 1 (3 volumes). Philadelphia: W. B. Saunders Company, 1973.

REFERENCES (CONTINUED)

Exercise 17

Basmajian, J. V. **Muscles Alive - Their Functions Revealed by Electromyography.** Baltimore: Williams and Wilkins Company, 1967.

Cromwell, L., Arditti, M., Weibell, F. J., Pfeiffer, E. A., Steele, B. and Labok, J. **Medical Instrumentation for Health Care.** Englewood Cliff, New Jersey: Prentice-Hall, Inc., 1976.

Lass, N. J. (Ed.). **Contemporary Issues in Experimental Phonetics.** New York: Academic Press, 1976.

Exercise 18

Kaplan, H. M. and Timmons, E. H. **The Rabbit: A Model for the Principles of Mammalian Physiology and Surgery.** New York: Academic Press, 1979.

Exercise 19

Darley, F. L. **Diagnosis and Appraisal of Communication Disorders. Englewood Cliffs,** New Jersey: Prentice-Hall, Inc., 1964.

Hamlet, S., Baker, D., Doudna, M., Hard, A. and Kumin, L. **Fundamentals of Hearing and Speech Science.** Columbus, Ohio: Collegiate Publishing Company, 1973.

Judson, L. S. V. and Weaver, A. T. **Voice Science.** 2nd edition. New York: Appleton-Century-Crofts, 1965.

Minifie, F. D., Hixon, T. J. and Williams, F.(Eds.). **Normal Aspects of Speech, Hearing and Language.** Englewood Cliffs, New Jersey: Prentice-Hall, Inc., 1973.

CHAPTER VI
Resonance

EXERCISE 20

VELOPHARYNGEAL ACTIVITY AND RESONANCE

OBJECTIVES

The student should gain knowledge of the structure of the soft palate, its movements for various speech sounds, and whether it has closure competency. The student should appreciate the meaning of resonance and its relation to wave motion.

TIME REQUIRED

One laboratory period - two or three hours

MATERIALS

Tongue depressors
Pen lights or standing lamps
Pharyngeal mirror
Glass straws
Matches

Pint bottles
Tuning forks
Burettes, used as columns (glass
  tubes)
Rubber tubing to fit the columns
Leveling bulbs

DESCRIPTION AND PROCEDURE

Structure and Movements of the Soft Palate

Direct a light into the oropharynx. Observe the position of the soft palate, the contours of the faucial pillars, the presence of scars, the size and color of the tonsils, and the relative dryness of the posterior pharyngeal wall. A tongue depressor facilitates visualization.

The nature of the movement of the velum and the related pharyngeal walls is very important. A simple procedure is to ask the subject to open his mouth, protrude his tongue, curl it down toward the chin, and voice a prolonged /E/ as in sEt, or an /i:/ as in bEEt. The normally active soft palate will lift vigorously. At this time the examiner should look for irregularities in palatal elevator action. If the phonemes above produce a tongue elevation that obliterates viewing the velum, test with /a/.

A further test of velopharyngeal closure is to ask the subject to produce a loud, prolonged /Θ/ sound (th). If he or she can accomplish this without nasal escape, this suggests potentially adequate closure.

Place a tongue depressor against the roof of the mouth and slide it posteriorly until it pushes the velum and produces a reflex response. Observe the degree of velar elevation with a mirror. Relate this to the action of the levator muscle of the palate. Does the entire velum including the uvula rise?

Other Functional Tests of Velopharyngeal Sufficiency

Have the subject undertake the "yawn" position, which involves raising the soft palate and lowering the back of the tongue. While he does this several times, observe the nature of the movements of the palate.

Have the subject pronounce vowel sounds and note whether his soft palate rises to touch the back wall of the pharynx.

Observe the nature of the velopharyngeal closure when the subject pronounces non-nasal English consonants.

Check the integrity of the subject's palate in the following actions:

Suck fluid through a straw.

Blow out a match held at some distance from the mouth.

Pronounce vowel sounds and sense whether they are unduly nasalized.
Note whether the voice has a muffled and obscure quality.
Observe whether the subject can sound the "stops" /p/, /b/, /t/,
/k/, /g/ for which the soft palate must be raised and the air passage
stopped at some point in the mouth.
Swallow forcibly. At the height of the action hold the position until
you have a definite kinesthetic consciousness of the action of the
velopharyngeal valve. Sense the pharyngeal action by holding your
hand at the angle of the mandible.

Pharyngeal (Gag) Reflex

Touch the back wall of the pharynx with a tongue depressor. The
pharyngeal muscles will contract, and gagging may occur. A positive
response indicates (in most people) normal functioning of cranial nerves IX and X.

Articulation Proficiency and Velopharyngeal Competence

In cleft palate V-P closure may be achieved in producing single
words, but not when contextual speech is used which requires exact
and rapid V-P adjustments. The comparison of proficiency between
single words and connected speech allows some estimation of V-P
competency in normal persons.

A test is presented below (Van Demark, 1964, By Permission) which
contains examples of fricatives, stop-plosives, glides, nasal
semivowels and blends which were created to approximate the
frequency of occurrence of the sounds found in the English language.
Have subjects repeat these sentences. Errors of stop-plosives and
fricatives and a predominance of distortion from too much nasal
emission point to faulty velopharyngeal closure.

> Most boys like to play football.
> Do you have a brother or sister?
> Ted had a dog with white feet.
> We shouldn't play in the street.
> Playing in the snow is fun.
> Nick's grandmother lives in the city.
> We go swimming on a very hot day.
> I like ice cream.

Tom has ham and eggs for breakfast.
We went to town yesterday.
Can you count to nine?
Do you want to take my new cap?
Do you know the name of my doll?

Some Tests of Nasal Emission

To determine that there is a free passage of breath through each nostril: The examiner says, "Observe what I do and repeat it." The examiner holds a piece of paper so that the upper right edge is positioned three inches away from his left nostril. Holding the right nostril closed with a finger of his right hand, he gently forces his breath through his left nostril for two seconds. If the breath stream is unimpeded, the upper right edge of the paper will be visibly blown. Similar directions should be followed for the right nostril.

To determine whether nasal resonance is involved in the production of non-nasal sounds, an assumption is made that the phonatory air normally escapes through the nose only during the articulation of the three nasal sounds, /m, n, ŋ/. The subject phonates a sentence none of whose sounds are nasal. (Ex: "What will you say if Jack goes to the circus?") During this, he holds a cold mirror in front of one nostril. This should become fogged only during the enunciation of a nasal sound.

To determine whether nasal resonance is withheld during the enunciation of nasal sounds, the subject says, "Now we will run for a long time." Because this includes several nasal sounds, there should be a nasal emission of breath on each nasal sound, accompanied by a film on the mirror. If there is no film, the subject has denasalized the sounds. (This test, if positive, suggests a high degree of hyporhinolalia; in mild cases a small film may show.)

It must be emphasized that any mirror test of nasal resonance presents a problem. Such tests may indicate air flow and not resonance. Air flow and resonance are two different events.

Feel the external nose with a finger. Vibrations will be felt during the enunciation of nasal sounds.

Resonance

Take a pint bottle with a small-sized neck and blow across its opening. Such a bottle gives off a tone of definite pitch. The air within has been caused to vibrate by being compressed and then rarefied. The pitch is proportional to the area of the opening and inversely proportional to the square root of the volume of the container. The vibratory movement of the air in the bottle is communicated to the air outside through the walls of the bottle and at the opening. The expanding air within produces compression of the air around the bottle and the outer air is set into vibratory movement.

Find a tuning fork which gives the same tone as the bottle, or by pouring the right quantity of water into it you can tune the bottle to the fork. When a vibrating fork is held over the mouth of a bottle, the natural tone of which is identical with that of the fork, the sound heard will be louder than that of the fork alone. The air in the bottle has been caused to vibrate at the same frequency as that of the fork. A fork of a different pitch will not cause this bottle to give off a tone unless its frequency is a multiple or sub-multiple of the other.

There are two ways thus to make the air in the bottle vibrate audibly. One is to excite it with air across its opening; the other is to impress upon the air in the bottle the vibrations of the tuning fork or the air around it which are of the frequency to which the cavity is resonant, or are of a frequency which is a multiple or submultiple of that frequency.

Hold a vibrating tuning fork over the mouth of the bottle. The energy forces the air in the bottle to vibrate in tune with the fork. Such vibrations are forced vibrations. The frequency of the free vibration of the air in the bottle is independent of the frequency of the air blown across its mouth; the frequency of the forced vibration is the frequency of the fork.

Resonance occurs when the frequency of the source which causes the forced vibrations is the same as the natural frequency of free vibrations of the system. The amplitude of the forced vibrations may be great. Resonant vibrations are a special case of forced vibrations. They have the frequency of the exciting source and they oscillate at their own natural frequency, the two frequencies being in this case the same.

Cavities have a range of resonance. A highly damped vibrating system responds to different frequencies; there is always one to which it responds most vigorously. This is the resonance frequency. A resonator may be broadly tuned. A sharply tuned resonator refuses to respond to vibrations out of tune with its resonance frequency by as little as one-tenth of one tone.

While holding a thin glass tumbler, tap it at its bottom. If the tumbler is held so that it cannot vibrate freely, the audible tone results from air vibrating inside the glass.

Place the mouth of the glass downward and tap it. Note the lowered pitch of the resonant tone. Bring the glass progressively nearer the palm of the hand by flexing the fingers and listen to the corresponding lower pitch of the tones when the glass is struck.

Explain the results in relation to the size of the opening and the changing volume of the cavity.

Velocity of Sound in Tubes

The velocity with which sound travels may be determined by multiplying frequency times wavelength.

The velocity of sound in air can be found by using a tuning fork of known frequency to produce a wave whose length will be measured by a resonating column of air (Figure 20-1).

The column is a glass tube, and its length is varied by changing the level of water in the tube. Resonance is indicated by the sudden increase in intensity of the sound when the column is adjusted to the proper length. Resonance occurs for different lengths of air column, and these lengths may be shown to be 1/4, 3/4, 5/4, etc. As the antinode is located a short distance out in the air, it is necessary to make a correction. This can be allowed for, if six-tenths of the radius of the tube is added to the length. This correction may be eliminated by subtraction of the resonance length of 1/4 λ from those for 3/4 λ, 5/4 λ, etc.

Fill the tube nearly full of water and mount a tuning fork of known frequency within a few millimeters of the top in such a manner that the prongs vibrate vertically. Start the fork vibrating by striking it with a hammer and slowly lower the water surface, listening for amplification of the note. When the proper length is obtained, a pronounced reinforcement of the sound will be audible. Make several

FIGURE 20-1
RESONANCE TUBE

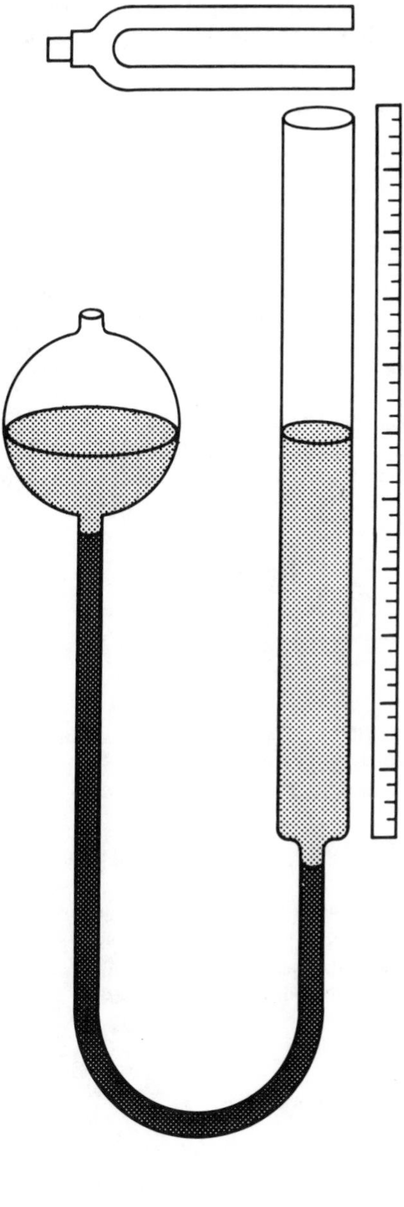

trials by running the water up and down. When the point of maximum intensity is located, mark the position of the water surface.

Lower the water and find the next resonance length. Continue as far as the length of the tube will permit. From the lengths of the different resonance chambers determine by subtraction the average value of the wavelength and calculate the velocity of sound at the existing temperature.

REVIEW

1. Explain how air columns of different lengths may produce resonance with the same note. Show why the length of the resonating column must, in the case studied, be an odd multiple of $1/4$. Is there a node or antinode at the closed end? At the open end?
2. Draw diagrams of the standing waves produced in the air column at each resonance length.
3. Using your determination of V_0, calculate the frequency of the fundamental and the first overtone of an open organ pipe 3 meters long. What would be the frequency of the fundamental and the first overtone of a closed pipe of the same length?

REFERENCES

Exercise 20

Emerick, L. L. and Hatten, J. T. **Diagnosis and Evaluation in Speech Pathology.** Englewood Cliffs, New Jersey: Prentice-Hall, Inc., 1974.

Judson, L. S. V. and Weaver, A. T. **Voice Science.** 2nd edition. New York: Appleton-Century-Crofts, 1965.

Ladefoged, P. **Elements of Acoustic Phonetics.** Chicago: University of Chicago Press, 1962.

Minifie, F. D., Hixon, T. J. and Williams, F. (Eds.), **Normal Aspects of Speech, Hearing and Language.** Englewood, N.J.: Prentice-Hall, Inc., 1973.

Van Demark, D. R. Misarticulations and Listener Judgments of Speech of Individuals with Cleft Palate. **Cleft Palate Journal.** 1:232-245, 1964.

CHAPTER VII
Articulation

EXERCISE 21

STRUCTURE AND ACTIONS OF ARTICULATORY ORGAN

OBJECTIVES

The student should ascertain the structure and the functional involvement of the major elements utilized in the articulation of vowels and consonants.

TIME REQUIRED

One laboratory period - two hours

Materials

Charts and models showing
    facial region in detail
Human skulls

Disarticulated human mandibles
    of various age groups

DESCRIPTION AND PROCEDURE

Lips

Refer back to Exercise 4 for procedures to observe the lip muscles and other muscles of facial expression. Many configurations of the lips are directed toward speech articulation. Utilizing charts and models, sketch the orbicularis oris muscle and the paired muscles inserting into it from above, laterally, and below.

Note the movements of the lips of your partner, as directed below. Can you observe facial movements for the muscles listed?

Elevating upper lip only	- Zygomaticus minor
	Levator labii superioris
	Levator labii superioris alaeque nasi
Depressing lower lip only	- Depressor labii inferioris
Approximating both lips	- Orbicularis oris
Protruding both lips	- Mentalis
	Deep fibers of orbicularis oris
Rounding the lips	- Orbicularis oris
Retracting the angles of the mouth	- Zygomaticus major
	Risorius
	Buccinator

Explain the physiologic effects of cleft lip. Consider the influence upon sounds which are dependent upon oral breath pressure. If the cleft is large, what might happen to /p/ and /b/?

Observe the interdependence of the articulators. As your subject moves his lips, note the simultaneous movements of the tongue and mandible. These actions occur in predictable sequences and they even affect the configurations of the pharynx and larynx.

Examples of Labial Involvement in Speech Sounds

Phonating certain labial consonants illustrates the part played by the lips. Produce the /p/ sound and analyze its anatomic correlates. The /p/ is a voiceless stop consonant. The /p/ is also a bilabial stop because the vocal tract is occluded at the lips. The same is true for /b/, except that /b/ is voiced. Bring to consciousness the kinesthetic sensation of the velum elevating in both of these sounds to minimize nasal emission.

Remember that allophones and phonemes are not uttered as isolated sounds. Both phonetic context and assimilation produce variations in these sounds and in the structural way they are produced.

Pathology of Lip Movement

The lips are active when articulating such labial consonants as /p, b, m/ and the labiodental consonants /f, v/. Labial distortions may not necessarily disturb the character of the sounds, however.

Observe on a subject the amount of labial tissue present and any apparent structural asymmetry. Are there evidences of a cleft?

Does the subject have any difficulty in approximating the lips and maintaining closure? Can he/she easily bring the lower lip to the upper teeth? Can each lip be moved independently?

Test the integrity of the facial nerve supply. Have the subject show his teeth, retract the mouth angles separately, and then both at one time, blow out the cheeks, purse the lips and whistle. If the subject smiles, does either side of the mouth show any droop? Do the lips have adequate motility? Have the subject repeat /pʌ/as in pUn for at least 5 seconds.

Tongue

Using charts and models, identify on them the root, corpus, apex, papillae and muscles of the tongue. Then locate the surface structures of the tongue dorsum in your laboratory partner.

Examine the tongue in activity in the subject. When the tongue is protruded, is it tremulous? Does it deviate markedly from the midline? Is it dry (indicating a subnormal hydration)? Is it smooth (indicating atrophy of papillae from some pathology)? Is it of expected size? What is its color? Color may change in disease, e.g. pink, salmon-colored, strawberry. Is the frenulum normal as contrasted with a short, thick, or abnormally attached frenulum? Have the subject pronounce several consonant and vowel phonemes, one at a time, and state the tongue muscles involved for each sound.

Kinesthetic Sensibility of the Tongue

Kinesthetic information allows appreciation of certain parameters of movement, i.e. bodily position and presence. The signals originate in mechanoreceptors located in joints (for the limbs) rather than in skeletal muscles and tendons. The systems are to be distinguished from (a) feedback mechanisms that begin in muscle and tendon spindles and give information about length or tension, and (b) receptors dealing with tactile competence (stereognosis). In strict terms, the tactile sense may be considered distinct from pain, temperature and the kinesthetic sense.

Curl the tip of your tongue behind the lower incisors. Force the tongue body and dorsum forward. Return the tongue to a resting position with its tip resting on the lower incisors. Repeat until you know that you have kinesthetic consciousness of the forward position of the tongue.

Involvement of the Tongue in Speech Sounds

The sound /Θ/ as in eTHer is a voiceless lingua-dental fricative. Observe the anatomy of its production by the tongue. Note that the tongue apex is placed against the back of the upper incisors, or against the cutting edge of those incisors, or between the upper and lower incisors. Then air is forced between the tongue apex and the place of contact. The soft palate can be felt to be raised to prevent nasal emission. Feel the larynx. Is there laryngeal vibration? Pronounce /ð/ as in eiTHer. Do you now feel laryngeal vibration? This sound is a voiced lingua-dental fricative.

Analyze the kinesiology of the sound /r/. When in front of a vowel, /r/ is a voiced fricative. Note that the tongue apex is raised toward the gum ridge, but does not contact the ridge. Palpate the larynx and sense the vibrations. Concentrate on the kinesthetic sensation that indicates the soft palatal elevation which prevents nasal emission of the sound.

Analyze the /ℓ/ sound. This is a voiced, lingua-alveolar consonant. Note that the tongue is raised so that its apex is in contact with the upper gum ridge. The tongue body behind the apex is relaxed and air escapes over the lateral aspect of the tongue. The middle of the tongue corpus is raised, its sides contacting the molars. Get the kinesthetic sensation of the elevation of the soft palate which prevents nasal emission of the sound.

Analyze the production of a nasal sound which also involves the tongue. Note in phonating /ŋ/ ng, a velar nasal continuant, that the back of the tongue contacts the lowered soft palate (which closes off the mouth). Palpate the larynx and sense the voiced vibrations.

The /s/ sound is important because it has a high degree of occurrence and because it is difficult to produce and is thus often distorted, as in lisping. In one acceptable manner of production, retract and slightly tense the lips, place the teeth in fairly close approximation, elevate the tongue and cup it to produce a depression along its median raphe, press the sides of the tongue along the inner edges of the gum as far forward as the central incisors, and raise the tongue toward the alveolar ridges. Sense that the velum is raised to prevent nasal emission of the sound.

It is emphasized that there are disagreements in points of view about the exact tongue postures described above.

Speed of Movement of the Tongue

Ask a subject to repeat the syllable /t ʌ/ (as in tUn) rapidly for at least 5 seconds, and note the speed of movement of the tongue tip. Have the subject sound /k ʌ/ for at least 5 seconds, and evaluate the motility and speed of the tongue root. Can you sense any disorders of rhythm in these sequences.

The tongue tip has the fastest movements of all the articulators. Its rate is 7.2 to 9.6 movements per second, the root movement being 5.4 to 8.9 (Hardcastle, 1976).

Rate of Oral Reading

Have a subject read a prose passage and record the reading time in seconds. Divide the number of words he reads (aloud) by the time involved. Multiply the quotient by 60 to convert the rate to words per minute. Compare the rates among all the members of your groups. It is to be noted that reading and speaking are different performances.

Mandible and Teeth

Examine disarticulated mandibles bearing teeth from skeletons of young adults. Compare the structure of mandibles and teeth from skeletons of young children and aged individuals. Note the number and condition of the natural and artificial teeth. What is the dental formula of the 32 permanent teeth? Study the alveolar sockets and describe their nerve and blood supply.

In skulls where both upper and lower teeth are fully present, can you draw any conclusions about the nature of the occlusion? What effects might occlusive malpositions have on speech? What is the classical Angle's classification of occlusions and malocclusions?

Mandibular Control

Draw schematically the nerve supply of the muscles of the mandible. Refer back to Exercise 4. List the muscles which contribute most to each of the following actions upon the mandible: elevation, depression, protrusion, retraction, and oblique lateral movement. These muscles are to be selected from the group: digastric, genioglossus, geniohyoid, masseter, mylohyoid, pterygoid external and internal, and temporal.

Refer back to Exercise 7 on cranial nerve testing. Test the integrity of the mandibular division of the trigeminal nerve and the temporal, masseter, and pterygoid muscles which the nerve supplies. With the subject tightly approximating his jaws, attempt to depress the mandible by pressing downward on his chin.

Have the subject slowly open his mouth and observe whether the mandible deviates to one side. This suggests weakness of the internal pterygoid muscle on that side.

Palate

Study in isolated skulls the bony details of the hard palate. For the soft palate (and its dependent muscular velum), use each person in your group as the subject. Is the velum length "normal," short, asymmetrical? Same for the uvula. What is the distance of the soft palate from the posterior wall of the pharynx in the "resting" (nonphonating) position? Is the palatal arch high, low or normal? Are the palatine tonsils present? What is their size? Their color?

Observe in the open mouth of a subject the three chief attachments of the velum: (1) anterior to the hard palate, (2) superior to the base of the skull, and (3) inferior to the tongue and pharynx. Are there only two modes of activity of the velum, the raising and lowering?

State which of the following muscles are elevators, depressors or tensors of the palate: levator palati, glossopalatal, pharyngopalatal, tensor palati and uvular muscle.

REFERENCES

Exercise 21

Bloomer, H. H. "Speech Defects Associated with Dental Malocclusion and Related Abnormalities." In L. E. Travis (Ed.). **Handbook of Speech Pathology and Audiology.** New York: Appleton-Century-Crofts, 1971, pp. 715-766.

Delp, M. H. and Manning, R. T. (Eds.). **Major's Physical Diagnosis.** 7th edition. Philadelphia: W. B. Saunders Company, 1968.

Fairbanks, G. **Voice and Articulation Drillbook.** 2nd edition. New York: Harper and Row, 1960.

Hardcastle, W. J. **Physiology of Speech Production.** New York: Academic Press, 1976.

Hopkins, H. U. **Leopold's Principles and Methods of Physical Diagnosis.** 3rd edition. Philadelphia: W. B. Saunders Comany, 1965.

Judge, R. D. and Zuidema, G.D. (Eds.). **Physical Diagnosis: A Physiologic Approach to the Clinical Examination.** 2nd edition. Boston: Little, Brown and Company, 1968.

Kampmeier, R. H. and Blake, T. M. **Physical Examination in Health and Disease.** 4th edition. Philadelphia: F. A. Davis Company, 1970.

Wheeler, R. C. **Dental Anatomy, Physiology and Occlusion.** 5th edition. Philadelphia: W. B. Saunders Company, 1974.

CHAPTER VIII
Ear and Hearing

EXERCISE 22

ANATOMY OF THE HUMAN EAR

OBJECTIVE

This study should give the student basic anatomic knowledge necessary to understand the transmission of sound waves throughout the ear.

TIME REQUIRED

One laboratory period - two hours

MATERIALS

Ear charts, disarticulated ossicles, models
Intact skeletons and intact skulls
Disarticulated temporal bones

Probes
Prosected temporal region, if there is availability to human cadavers

DESCRIPTION AND PROCEDURE

External Ear

Pinna

Identify the landmarks on the pinna of your laboratory partner. The pinna is surrounded by a rim called the helix. Inside the helix is a parallel prominence, the antihelix. Between the helix and antihelix posteriorly, the scaphoid fossa ends inferiorly in the lobule, or ear lobe. Sketch the pinna and draw in muscles related to it. Refer to Figure 22-1.

FIGURE 22-1
PINNA OF EAR

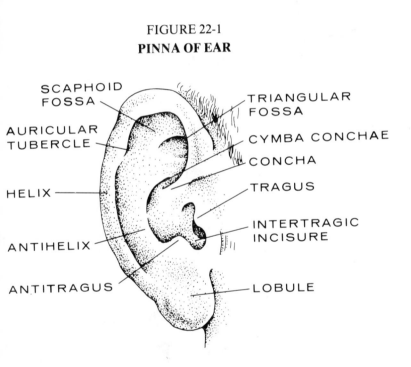

By moving a finger from the front to the external canal, one pushes a cartilage continuation of the pinna called the tragus over the opening. The tragus is opposed by a flap called the antitragus. A depression, the concha, runs into the external canal. The concha is seen posteriorly between the mid-antihelix and the external canal.

External Auditory Canal

With an otoscope, and only under supervision of an audiologist or otologist, examine the external auditory canal of your subject. If the medial aspect of the ear is relatively free of wax, note the topographical regions and surface landmarks of the tympanic membrane. Well illustrated anatomic textbooks should be available.

Temporal Bone

Examine disarticulated temporal bones. Refer back to Exercise 3 and also to atlases and textbooks of anatomy. Identify all parts of this important bone.

On the intact skull, observe the relationships of the temporal bone to adjacent bones. What is the nature of the articulations?

Middle Ear

Ossicles

Examine models containing the ear ossicles to visualize their shapes, relative positions, and actions. Refer to Figures 22-2 and 22-3.

FIGURE 22-2

CORONAL SECTION OF EAR

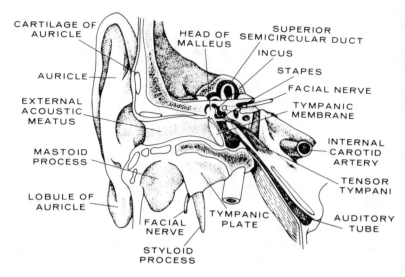

FIGURE 22-3
MIDDLE EAR

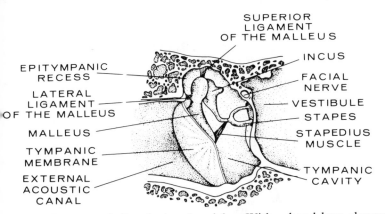

Examine natural disarticulated ossicles. With a hand lens observe their articular surfaces. Describe the movements that occur at their joints.

Auditory Tube

Using an intact skull, locate the position of the auditory tube. Describe from charts the muscles that are intimately related to it along its length. What is its primary closing muscle?

The eponym, Eustachian (eustachian) tube, should preferably be supplanted by the term, auditory tube.

Describe how closing your nose and mouth while exhaling would help to open a stuffed ear in a descending airplane.

State the mechanisms in the middle ear which are protective against loud noises.

Internal Ear

Draw a diagram of an uncoiled cochlea, showing the oval window, round window, and the canals and vibrating membranes. Draw a cross-section of the cochlea, labelling its parts. Label regions of the basilar membrane responding to an increasing succession of sound pitches.

Find all parts implied in the above on models, charts and prepared skulls. Figure 22-2 is a coronal section of the entire ear. Figure 22-4 displays the labyrinth as a whole.

FIGURE 22-4
LABYRINTH

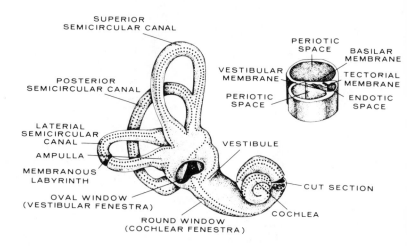

EXERCISE 23

TUNING FORK TESTS AND AUDIOMETRY

OBJECTIVES

The student should obtain an understanding of many tests of auditory function including the evaluation of auditory sensitivity. The present Exercise provides an extremely limited introduction and students cannot be expected to apply the procedures to clinical situations until they have undergone training in audiometry and audiology and are professionally competent. Both tuning fork tests and pure tone audiometer tests are included herein.

TIME REQUIRED

One laboratory period - at least two hours

MATERIALS

Pure tone audiometer   Tuning forks   256, 512, 1024 Hz

DESCRIPTION

Tuning fork tests have been used extensively in the past to help distinguish perception from transmission deafness (a better term being loss of hearing). These tests still have value in understanding some medical reports. They are noninvasive and simple to perform. Their interpretation in diagnosis, however, is a matter for expert opinion and they have been superseded except in special circumstances by audiometry.

Miller (1979) discusses the present value of tuning fork tests in terms of their usefulness versus the current widespread view that they are inconsistent and unreliable. Miller claims that the audiometer does not completely replace the tuning fork in auditory testing.

The pure tone audiometer has been the most widely used basic instrument for testing hearing. The present Exercise utilizes the audiometer for two air conduction tests. One is a screening test called a sweep check and the other evaluates the hearing threshold for several frequencies.

PROCEDURE

Tuning Fork Tests

Rinne's Test

This test helps in the decision as to whether conductive hearing loss is present. Sound a tuning fork and hold it in front of the ear to be tested with the points close to and in line with the external auditory meatus. Ask the subject frequently if the tuning fork is heard. As soon as he stops hearing the tuning fork, transfer it to his mastoid process. If it is not heard there, reverse the procedure. If the tuning fork is heard by air conduction after it is heard by bone conduction, Rinne's test is said to be positive (normal). If it is heard when the fork is transferred to the mastoid process, after it has stopped being heard by air, the bone conduction is said to be better than air conduction, and Rinne's test is negative. If the test is positive, there is apparently no marked degree of conductive hearing loss.

Weber's Test

This test is used for comparing degrees of hearing loss in two ears, both of which are affected in the same way. It depends on the fact that in conductive loss, bone conduction is better than air conduction. Sound a tuning fork and place it on the midline of the forehead. Ask the subject in which ear the sound is best heard. In conductive hearing loss in one ear, the subject can be expected to point to that ear as the one in which the sound is heard best. If both ears are affected by a conductive loss, the tuning fork should be heard best in the one which is more obstructed. In sensori-neural loss, assuming that the middle ear is normal, the sound is conveyed entirely by bone conduction and will be heard best on the side which has the better functioning nerve (that is, the ear with less hearing loss will hear the tuning fork).

Schwabach's Test

This test has a twofold purpose: to indicate sensori-neural hearing loss not only where it is the sole cause of a hearing impairment, but also to find the underlying degree of sensori-neural loss in persons who suffer from a conductive loss. Perform the test by sounding a tuning fork and placing it on the mastoid process of a subject. When the subject stops hearing the tuning fork, transfer the fork to your own mastoid process. If you as the examiner can hear the tuning fork, the Schwabach test on the subject is said to be shortened. The test presupposes perfect hearing by the examiner. A modification of the Schwabach test, called Absolute Bone Conduction, compares the length of time which the subject hears the tuning fork placed on the mastoid process with the time length heard by the examiner. In a conductive loss, the length of time the subject hears the fork is longer than that of the examiner; in a perceptive loss, it is shorter.

Pure Tone Audiometry for Hearing Sensitivity

Air Conduction Threshold
1. First become familiar with the audiometer. Turn on the power switch
2. With phones on your own ears, ascertain the sensation when manipulating the intensity control.
3. Locate the control that switches the signal between phones. Send the signal to each phone in turn, change the intensity and feel the sensation
4. Go up and down the pitch range with the frequency control. Switch the signal to your other ear and repeat the procedure.
5. Determine the function of the interrupter switch. The tone is transmitted through the phones only by depressing this switch.

Give directions to the subject as follows: You will hear tones, some high and others low in pitch. Some tones will be faint and others loud. Signal by raising your hand when you hear a tone. Put your hand down when the tone disappears.

After removing the subject's eyeglasses if worn, place the earphones on him and determine an air conduction threshold for 250, 500, 1000, 2000 and 4000 Hz.

1. Start at 1000 Hz where there is good responsiveness.
2. Unless the subject activates the interrupter switch, assume that he does not hear the signal. For every successive frequency tested, start with the intensity level minimal. Activate the interrupter switch and increase the tone intensity until it is audible to the subject. Add an additional 20 dB for ease of hearing, except for very sensitive subjects.
3. By working the intensity control, decrease the intensity level until hearing becomes lost. Note this point.
4. Increase the intensity until hearing is just restored. Note this point. The procedure brackets the threshold fairly narrowly.
5. Release the interrupter and the subject should not hear a tone. Upon depressing the interrupter, check whether the tone is heard. If not, go directly to step 7.
6. If the tone is heard, release the interrupter switch and drop the intensity by 10 dB. The tone should not be heard.

7. Discontinue the tone, increase the intensity by 5 dB and depress the interrupter. This step can be repeated if a higher intensity is necessary for audibility.
8. Release the interrupter and drop the intensity by 10 dB. At this level, a tone should not be heard. If it is heard, repeat step 8 to a point of inaudibility.
9. Increase the intensity by 5 dB and depress the interrupter. If the tone is inaudible, increase the intensity another 5 dB, depress the interrupter and continue to a point of audibility. At this level decrease the intensity by 10 dB and present tones at 5 dB steps of increasing intensity until audibility occurs. At threshold decrease the intensity. Repeat this procedure several times. The threshold is the lowest hearing level at which there is correct response at least 50 per cent of the time.

Repeat the testing for 250, 500, 1000 (to recheck), 2000, 4000 and 1000 Hz (for doublecheck). Construct an audiogram. Test the other ear, repeating all procedures.

Sweep Check Screening Test

This test is a screening procedure to find whether hearing is within a normal range.

1. Introduce a 500 Hz tone, at 30 dB, into one ear. If the tone is heard, release the interrupter switch and set the intensity at 20 dB.
2. Introduce the 20 dB tone enough times to know whether the subject is hearing that intensity tone. Then test at 1000, 2000, 4000 and 6000 Hz. If there is no response at 500 or 4000 Hz, increase the intensity to 25 dB and retest 500 and 4000.
3. Switch the tone to the other ear and repeat the test, starting with 6000 Hz and descending.

REFERENCES

Exercise 22

Anderson, J. E. **Grant's Atlas of Anatomy.** 7th edition. Baltimore: Williams and Wilkins Comapny, 1978.

Keidel, W. D. and Neff, W. D. (eds.). **Handbook of Sensory Physiology. V/1. Auditory System.** New York: Springer-Verlag, 1974.

Minifie, F. D., Hixon, T. J. and Williams, F. (Eds.). **Normal Aspects of Speech, Hearing and Language.** Englewood Cliffs, New Jersey: Prentice-Hall, 1973.

Paparella, M. M. and Shumrick, D. A. (Eds.). **Otolaryngology.** Volume 1 (3 volumes). Philadelphia: W. B. Saunders Company, 1973.

Spalteholz, W. and Spanner, R. **Atlas of Human Anatomy.** 16th edition. Philadelphia: F. A. Davis Company, 1961.

Warwick, R. and Williams, P. L. **Gray's Anatomy.** 16th edition. Philadelphia: W. B. Saunders Company, 1980.

Exercise 23

Fulton, R. T. and Lloyd, L. L. **Auditory Assessment of the Difficult-to-Test.** Baltimore: Williams and Wilkins Company, 1975.

Langenbeck, B. **Textbook of Practical Audiometry.** Baltimore: Williams and Wilkins Company, 1965.

Miller, G. W. Tuning Fork Decay. **Laryngoscope** 89(3):459-472, 1979.

Newby, H. A. **Audiology.** New York: Appleton-Century-Crofts, 1972.

Index

#461
L.H